GUARDING THE GOLDEN GATE

GUARDING *THE* GOLDEN GATE

A History of the US Quarantine Station in San Francisco Bay

J. Gordon Frierson, MD

UNIVERSITY OF NEVADA PRESS | *Reno & Las Vegas*

University of Nevada Press | Reno, Nevada 89557 USA
www.unpress.nevada.edu
Cover photograph courtesy of the California History Room, California State Library,
Sacramento, California.

LIBRARY OF CONGRESS CATALOGING-IN-PUBLICATION DATA
Names: Frierson, J. Gordon (John Gordon), 1935– author.
Title: Guarding the Golden Gate : a history of the US Quarantine Station in San Francisco
    Bay / J. Gordon Frierson.
Description: Reno : University of Nevada Press, [2022] | Includes bibliographical references
    and index.
Summary: "Amidst the evolving scientific knowledge of epidemic diseases during the
    mid-to-late nineteenth century, Guarding the Golden Gate narrates the development of the
    quarantine station on Angel Island in the San Francisco Bay and illuminates the everyday
    activities of the station's personnel as they met both political and public health challenges."
    —Provided by publisher.
Identifiers: LCCN 2021041543 | ISBN 9781647790462 (paperback) | ISBN 9781647790479 (ebook)
Subjects: LCSH: San Francisco Quarantine Station (Angel Island, Calif.)—History. |
    Quarantine—California—Angel Island—History. | San Francisco Bay (Calif.)—History.
Classification: LCC RA667.C2 F75 2022 | DDC 614.4/6097946—dc23 LC record available at,
    https://lccn.loc.gov/2021041543

The paper used in this book meets the requirements of American National Standard for
Information Sciences—Permanence of Paper for Printed Library Materials, ANSI/NISO
Z39.48-1992 (R2002).

FIRST PRINTING

Manufactured in the United States of America

To Veska, with love.

Contents

Illustrations follow page 62.

Introduction

San Francisco Bay is one of the most striking in the world. Formed by the outpouring of sixteen rivers flowing down from the Sierra Nevada, it covers about four hundred square miles within an undulating shoreline. Its waters course to the Pacific Ocean through a relatively narrow passage, flanked on each side by imposing bluffs, known as the "Golden Gate." In the years before 1848, traffic through the Golden Gate was sparse. Beautiful as it was, there was little within the Bay to attract visitors arriving by sea.

This peaceful state of affairs changed, though, as news of the discovery of gold in the California hills flew around the globe. Soon thousands of frenzied visitors passed between the bluffs in a rush for riches. The stampede of fortune-seekers transformed San Francisco from a sleepy village into a bustling city. A decade or two later, as the allure of gold waned, newer immigrants descended the gangplanks of incoming vessels to seek work on railroads, in farming, and in other enterprises. San Francisco absorbed the newcomers and grew rapidly, assisted in no small part by its accessible harbor.

The accelerating numbers of ships from Asian and South American harbors inevitably brought a few passengers who had sickened on the way. Some suffered from diseases such as smallpox and cholera, maladies that were prevalent in many ports and were feared in California. Efforts to keep epidemic diseases from stepping ashore in San Francisco included the institution of quarantine measures. Quarantine, defined as the holding in isolation of persons suffering from, or exposed to, contagious disease for a period of time until the danger of transmitting the disease has passed, was an old practice and a feature of most busy ports.

This book tells the story of the US quarantine station on Angel Island in San Francisco Bay: the Angel Island Quarantine Station. At the time the Station opened, 1891, diseases such as smallpox, cholera, yellow fever, typhus, and plague ravaged various parts of the globe. Before the modern era of antibiotics and vaccinations, these scourges, if brought by

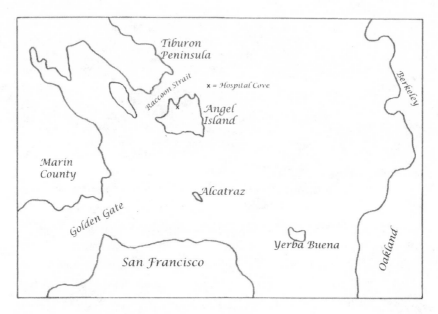

San Francisco Bay Area, showing major landmarks present when the station opened.

arriving ship passengers, posed imminent threats to San Francisco's population. The atmosphere of fear was heightened by the fact that the scientific world knew little about how epidemic diseases were transmitted. Isolation of sick people, however, seemed a sensible way to prevent spread. Consequently, health officials searched for a site where new arrivals with contagious disease, and those exposed to them, could be removed from contact with the general population and undergo a period of quarantine. An island provided the ideal setting.

Several islands lie scattered in the Bay. One of the larger ones, Angel Island, is easily visible about two miles north of San Francisco. Its location, size, and accessibility rendered it suitable as a site for a quarantine station. Eventually, the federal government acquired land on the island, built the quarantine station, and assigned the Marine Hospital Service (MHS), a service that had recently assumed quarantine responsibilities for the nation, to operate it. The design of the quarantine facility followed emerging concepts in medicine and public health that were still evolving and incomplete by 1891. Political maneuvering and the pressures of commerce also exerted significant influence on the development of the Station.

The story begins, interestingly, in New Orleans. Long before the gold rush, outbreaks of yellow fever had battered New Orleans almost every summer. In a search for protection from the repeated visitations and even though the medical world was still in the dark about how the disease spread, public health officers devised an elaborate quarantine technique. Because the new procedures proved effective (most of the time), the New Orleans quarantine system became a model for other ports around the nation, including San Francisco.

Quarantine services are sometimes confused with immigration services. They were, and are, separate and distinct. The US Immigration Service did indeed maintain a station on Angel Island, not far from the quarantine station, but it did not open until 1910, nineteen years after the quarantine station began operations. The two services operated independently, under different branches of government. The quarantine service carried out an initial inspection of immigrants looking for evidence of specific epidemic diseases, and conducted a cleansing of ships, luggage, clothing, and the passengers themselves. Only then did they hand passengers over to immigration personnel who would determine, following immigration law, acceptability for entry into the United States. Officers of the quarantine service also performed medical examinations for the Immigration Service as an aid in their evaluations for entry but made no independent decisions about entry or rejection. Experiences at the Immigration Station have generated much literature focused on the tensions, poor conditions, and psychological burdens suffered by detained immigrants. The prolonged harassment experienced by many was not a feature of quarantine. The quarantine facilities were undeniably rustic and racial prejudices darkened the quarantine experience, but undergoing the process was a brief event for most and lasted up to a few weeks for the remainder.

The opening of the quarantine station coincided with an age when people traveling across oceans, along coastlines, and even across continents reached their destinations by ship or sailing vessel. At the same time, cholera, smallpox, plague, and other scourges loomed ominously around much of the globe. Motor vehicles, electric power, telephones, and public health measures such as sewerage and clean water were nonexistent or in early stages of development. On Angel Island the first quarantine crews worked in grassy, fire-prone surroundings devoid of telephones, electricity, adequate water, and schools. As the nineteenth century drew to a close, scientific knowledge was advancing rapidly. The discovery that tiny germs caused disease had initiated a revolution in medical thought.

Contagious and febrile diseases could now be diagnosed accurately, even if their treatment persisted as a challenge. Working out how germs passed from one person to another, a central issue in quarantine work, was a later achievement. When the first quarantine officers arrived at the Station, they operated with an incomplete understanding of disease transmission. The subsequent adaptation of procedures at Angel Island to evolving medical knowledge of epidemic disease is a central feature of quarantine history.

When the Station opened, San Francisco was unlike the city of today. It was emerging from its recent turbulent history of gold fever, pioneering railroads, and outsized personalities. The refinements of cultural life were emerging, business interests were a dominant force, and scrappy newspapers exerted exceptional influence. Booming trade and new wealth perhaps gave the residents an inflated self-confidence. Always, though, the menace of plagues from abroad was dimly perceptible, despite attempts to ignore it.

The story of the Angel Island Quarantine Station is a journey through San Francisco history and the history of medical thought, with its measures of stress, uncertainty, and hard labor, yet enriched with periods of inspiration and progress.

GUARDING THE GOLDEN GATE

CHAPTER ONE

Death in the Hold

LATE IN THE DAY ON MAY 6, 1882, a British-owned three-hundred-foot steamship slowed its engines as it approached San Francisco Bay. The vessel, the SS *Altonower*, built for the cargo trade only two years earlier, had been diverted from activity in the Indian Ocean to take advantage of an unusual situation, a sudden demand to accommodate large numbers of Chinese seeking passage from their homeland to San Francisco. The *Altonower* responded to the call and before long was bearing in its hull a human cargo of 829 passengers, mainly impoverished and poorly educated Chinese from the southeastern area of the Qing Empire. The journey had been a long one. After leaving Hong Kong, the vessel had made a brief stop in Yokohama, Japan, and finally had motored for eighteen tedious days across the Pacific Ocean.

The *Altonower* steered its way through the windswept bluffs overlooking the north and south boundaries of the narrow passage into San Francisco Bay, a passage known locally as the Golden Gate. The soldier-explorer John Fremont had bestowed the name because it reminded him of the entrance to the Golden Horn, a narrow strait adjacent to Istanbul. The passengers assembled on deck surveyed the shoreline as the ship drifted by, gleaning the first impressions of their new home. Below, in a hold constructed for cargo and devoid of portholes, others sensed the arrival by the diminished engine noise and excited comments from above. The more curious scrambled up to catch their first glimpse of San Francisco Bay, a four-square-mile body of water tucked in behind the Gate. Directly ahead, the vessel approached the rocky, windswept, and barren island of Alcatraz, which in later years would be home to a notorious prison. Farther to the left and close to the northern shore of the Bay rose the hills of Angel Island, a larger, less-rocky, grass-covered landmass partly obscuring the view beyond. A variety of craft dotted the water: sailing vessels of various sizes, steamships, ferries, fishing boats, and the occasional Chinese junk. As Alcatraz slipped by the ship on the left, to the right the bustling city of San Francisco came into view, its houses and buildings clinging to the rising coast. From the shore multiple piers, alive with activity, jutted into the Bay. On the piers were containers of silks, piles of lumber, and crates of numerous foods. Meiggs Wharf, the largest of them, built by the failed entrepreneur Henry Meiggs to accommodate lumber ships, was unmistakable in its L-shape and estimated two-thousand-foot length. The *Altonower*'s passengers, all men leaving grinding poverty at home, absorbed the novel sights as they contemplated their life ahead.

Ironically, on the day that the *Altonower* arrived, three thousand miles away in Washington, DC, President Chester A. Arthur was putting his pen to legislation prohibiting the immigration of just the sort of Chinese people the ship carried: common laborers. For months, politicians in Washington had been debating legislation on the exclusion of Chinese, especially laborers. The final product, the Chinese Exclusion Act, took effect ninety days after the president appended his signature. The news of the impending legislation had reached thousands of miles to the land targeted by the bill, where it precipitated a rush of Chinese to reach American shores before the gates closed. The 829 passengers on the Altonower were only a small portion of an unprecedented surge in Chinese immigration, people who were scrambling to reach the United States, especially California, before the deadline.

The Exclusion Act specifically prohibited the immigration of Chinese laborers, defined as "both skilled and unskilled laborers and Chinese employed in mining."[1] Students, merchants, diplomatic personnel, travelers, and their dependents fell outside the definition of laborer, constituting a small group still allowed to enter the country. Chinese already resident in the United States retained the right to leave and return as desired, though they needed certain papers to do so, and Chinese were barred from becoming American citizens.[2] Once the bill became law it would be impossible, with the exceptions mentioned above, for a Chinese person to immigrate or, if already a resident in the country, to bring over family members.

In earlier years the lure that attracted Chinese, and others, to California was Gum Shan, the Cantonese expression for Gold Mountain. In January 1848 the discovery of gold in the American River, not far from Sacramento, precipitated a rush of fortune hunters from around the world. Driven by visions of fast wealth, the gold seekers arrived in droves by land and sea from all parts of America and abroad. Before long a vast forest of masts sprang up along the San Francisco shore, marking the vessels abandoned by crews eager for their piece of the lustrous metal. From this raucous, disorganized beginning, the city of San Francisco emerged, prospered, and matured shakily as it added new businesses and civic government. By 1882 it was the largest city and port on the west coast, with a population of just over a quarter of a million people.

Most Chinese who had originally sought their fortune at Gold Mountain found themselves edged out of gold mining through various discriminatory actions, and they drifted into other areas of employment. One major activity, requiring thousands of workers, was the construction of the Central Pacific Railroad, the western end of the first transcontinental railroad. As the years passed, and after release from railroad work, the Chinese settled into other occupations. Before long they constituted 50 to 75 percent of the farm labor of the state, provided ongoing labor for new railroads, dominated the boot and shoe industries in San Francisco, and were major players in cigar manufacturing, laundries, and other areas.[3] Between 1870 and 1880, 138,941 Chinese had immigrated to the United States, primarily to California, and the numbers showed no sign of slowing.[4] Their situation became more precarious in the 1870s when a financial depression created job scarcity and consequent political pressure to restrict Chinese immigration. The harassment from California, combined with hostility to Chinese immigration in other parts of the country, came together in the form of the Chinese Exclusion Act.[5]

Though life for the Chinese in California was difficult, those in China wrestled with far greater suffering. Bureaucratic corruption, interruptions of food transport, spreading opium addiction, and several popular uprisings brought uncertainty and hardship. The subsequent violent civil wars of the Taiping Rebellion devastated the country, uprooting families, destroying homes, and shattering the economy.[6] Recovery was slow, and existence was especially arduous in Guangdong Province, where most of the recent immigrants originated. Life in California remained a powerful attraction.

Immigration numbers mounted quickly. At the end of February 1882, the *San Francisco Chronicle* reported that 8,468 Chinese had arrived that month, compared with only 300 in February 1881, and that the numbers were continuing to rise.[7] The total for 1882 up to the date of the Exclusion Act was 39,579 immigrants.[8] Steamship companies that did not usually ply the China-Japan–San Francisco route suddenly rushed in, eager for the extra passenger business. Freighters that were converted in slipshod fashion to carry human cargo, usually referred to as tramp steamers and often lacking proper ventilation and reasonable cleanliness, became commonplace in the Bay. At times, they carried passengers packed in beyond the legal limits and incurred significant fines. Congress, in attempts to render steerage class conditions tolerable if not comfortable, enacted various laws addressing space, food, and ventilation, with the latest being the Passenger Act of 1882.[9] Nevertheless, ships still emerged from shipyards with areas of their hulls designated for "Cargo or Steerage Passengers," a sign of the conditions of steerage class. The *Altonower* was one of the tramp steamers, although the circumstances below deck did not violate the Passenger Act.

As the ship eased past the San Francisco shoreline, the crew threw the anchor near Black Point, a bulge in the shoreline now known as Fort Mason Recreational Park. The next day the Quarantine Officer boarded the vessel to inspect for the presence of a quarantinable disease. At the time, five diseases qualified as quarantinable: smallpox, plague, cholera, yellow fever, and typhus. Smallpox was the most worrisome, and eighty-five passengers with smallpox had already been removed that year from other incoming vessels, in spite of an increasing number being vaccinated during the previous two years.[10] (A policy of compulsory vaccination on board ship had gone into effect two years earlier in response to a request from the San Francisco Health Department.)[11]

After boarding the *Altonower,* the Quarantine Officer unearthed disturbing information: Shortly after leaving Yokohama, the ship's medical officer (often called the surgeon) had attempted to vaccinate the passengers against smallpox. But when the doctor prepared to administer the vaccine, he faced a simmering mutiny. One passenger, in particular, posted signs in the hold claiming that the procedure was poisonous and rallied his compatriots to protest. The doctor, afraid for his safety, abandoned the effort and the captain acquiesced, considering his crew unprepared to put down a mutiny.[12]

Smallpox was a worrisome disease. A viral infection spread primarily through the respiratory route, it was particularly contagious in enclosed spaces, exacting a mortality rate of around 30 percent. Viral particles spewed out from a cough, sneeze, or even conversation easily infected others close by. Vaccination was a safe, preventive measure, unfortunately neglected during the fateful journey of the *Altonower.* Smallpox was, furthermore, no stranger to San Francisco. Outbreaks rattled the city in 1868–69, 1872–73, and 1876–77, the latter producing more than 1,600 cases.[13] Blame for outbreaks often focused on the Chinese, both the recent arrivals by ship and those residing in San Francisco's overcrowded Chinatown.[14] In the year before the *Altonower* arrived, the virus struck again, afflicting 507 residents.[15] The Health Officer's report that year included a plea for a proper quarantine facility, a place on shore where incoming passengers exposed to disease could be watched in isolation and treated if needed.[16] The plea drew no response.

On the *Altonower* the unvaccinated passengers faced the Quarantine Service rule requiring vaccination, by force if necessary, before disembarking. A similar situation two months earlier on the SS *Suez*, whose surgeon had also abandoned vaccination in the face of death threats, set the tone. The *Suez*'s captain brought the 577 Chinese passengers up on deck and herded them to the stern, closed the hatches and gangways, and stationed armed men at strategic points. A newspaper report reflects vividly the prejudicial anti-Chinese tone of the time:

> The first one secured was a large, muscular Mongolian, with the instincts of a Tartar. No sooner had he been secured than a whole band of his frightened and half-frenzied followers raised a cry that was heard distinctly by workmen on the seawall, about a mile away. They rushed forward and attempted to break down the barricades but were driven back by the determined men who stood on guard. Force had to be used and was used with disastrous effect upon the faces of several of the ringleaders. The man who had been secured as the first victim fought like a demon and seemed determined not to be subdued. Four strong men were required to drag him through the passageway and hold him firmly to the deck while Dr. McAllister (the Quarantine Officer) performed the dreaded operation…The next five or six had to be secured in like manner and resisted to the end as if expecting nothing less than decapitation.[17]

Resistance gradually died down and the entire group submitted to vaccination. The printed lines exuded animosity to the Chinese, a common refrain in the newspapers.

A similar scene played out on the *Altonower*. The wary passengers were clustered on the afterdeck, their sleeves rolled up, guards posted, and compulsory vaccination begun. A drop of virus-containing liquid was placed on the upper arm and scratched into the superficial skin with a small needle. The recalcitrant ringleaders struggled at first and some attempted to suck up the residual vaccine fluid as they descended to quarters below, but the remainder submitted without incident. The crew had already been vaccinated.

The Quarantine Officer was not finished. As a further measure to ensure that no residual smallpox germs remained, he planned a fumigation of the *Altonower*. On the following day, when he informed the assembled passengers through an interpreter that poisonous chlorine gas was to be pumped into the ship's hold, a few passengers became visibly agitated, gesticulating urgently. They reluctantly admitted the presence of a stowaway in the hold, too ill to come up. The surgeon descended into the windowless hull and located the emaciated victim, hot with fever, and heavily covered with telltale pox. He was removed and taken by horse-drawn ambulance to the city's smallpox hospital on Twenty-Sixth Street, known locally as the Pesthouse. The crew hoisted the traditional yellow flag, signifying quarantine, fumigated the hold with chlorine, and washed the rest of the ship with disinfectant.[18] The stowaway died in the Pesthouse a few days later.

The smallpox victim was off the ship but the damage had been done. The Quarantine Officer imposed the mandatory two-week quarantine on the remaining passengers, who remained on board ship since there was no facility on shore for them. Held captive in cramped quarters, it was only a few days before scattered individuals felt the heat of fever, the pain of headache, and watched as small, fluid-filled bumps (called vesicles), the dreaded pox, developed on the skin. Full immunity from the recent vaccination would not take effect for ten days or so. In the meantime, the virus from the stowaway could make its way through the confined passengers.

At first, only a few became ill, and they were duly removed to the Pesthouse. Then the numbers exploded. On the tenth day after arrival, the surgeon diagnosed forty-two passengers with active smallpox, all needing medical care. To put them ashore, the crew herded the entire group of forty-two into two of the ship's lifeboats, twenty-six in the first and sixteen in the second, while a third boat, carrying crew members, acted as escort. A rope connected the three boats in a line as the steam launch maneuvered to tow them ashore. The wind that day was strong and gusty and the sea rough. As the launch veered toward the city, the lifeboats swung broadside to the heightened surf. Spray swept over the gunwales and waves rocked the lifeboats wildly. In the boat of sixteen, several Chinese panicked and stood up, capsizing the vessel, and catapulting the smallpox-ridden passengers into the cold waters. The crew on the launch reacted quickly, hurling out life preservers and lowering another lifeboat. Clinging to the capsized hull only eight Chinese were visible. A rapid search disclosed seven more under the overturned boat. The fifteen were hoisted exhausted and shivering onto the steam launch, driven to shore, and admitted to the Pesthouse. A long and careful search failed to find the one missing passenger.

Meanwhile, hundreds of Chinese on the deck of the *Altonower* watched the action closely and somehow assumed that the capsize was deliberate, an attempt to drown the sick passengers. Enraged, and no doubt terrified, they threw the doctor's chair overboard, grabbed whatever weapons they could find—sledgehammers, capstans, axes—and charged after the captain, officers, and the already-hated ship's surgeon. Flag signals of distress went up as the panic-stricken officers barricaded themselves inside a cabin, fearing they would not emerge alive. But the distress signals were recognized, and before long a police launch arrived and restored order. The ship's doctor was so shaken that he refused to venture into the hold to look for further smallpox cases. Instead, he made inspections on deck, with guards present.[19] The corpse of the missing Chinese passenger turned up the next day, floating near shore.

At this point, the smallpox hospital, with space for fifty-two patients, was full. The city refused to allow more sufferers to land unless the steamship company agreed to reimburse the extra expenses, including those that might be incurred in case smallpox spread beyond the Pesthouse. The owners of the *Altonower*, Adams Bros. of London, demurred, saying that the ship had been leased to a firm in Hong Kong and that firm had the responsibility. The chartering firm, Russell & Company, through their local representative, Macondray & Company, insisted at first that they were not responsible, but soon backtracked and began seeking a location with isolation facilities. They turned to the established lines, the Pacific Mail (PMSS) Steamship Company and the Occidental and Oriental (O&O) Steamship Company. These companies already had chartered ships outfitted to accommodate passengers in case of quarantine, but they declined to make them available. Building a shed on the Bay's northern shore was suggested but rejected since local residents refused to live near smallpox.

Other attempts to find suitable quarantine facilities failed. Further squabbling over expenses and the safety of alternate vessels dragged on as if time did not matter.[20] Meanwhile, the passengers remained imprisoned on the *Altonower*. The chartering company did agree to reimburse the city for any further cases sent to the Pesthouse, though the rumor floated that reimbursement was not likely to happen. The ship's agents denied this.[21]

The virus marched on within the *Altonower*'s hold, hunting down one after another of the passengers, sometimes as many as seven to ten in one day. By June 4, twenty-nine days after arrival, a total of eighty-four passengers had taken ill, and three or four had perished.[22] The low mortality rate suggests that the vaccinations were offering partial protection after the first few days.

The local Chinese consul-general, Frederick Bee, had been following events and was outraged at the needless suffering. Bee, born in Clinton, New York, was studying for a law degree when news of gold in California reached him, impelling him to try his luck out West. He found, though, that he preferred business to mining; he settled in San Francisco and went into business. While in the gold country, he had witnessed discriminatory practices inflicted on the Chinese and developed a sympathy for their plight. Over time he used his legal skills to become, in effect, a lawyer for local Chinese and defended their interests until his death. In 1876 he defended Chinese concerns before a congressional committee meeting in San Francisco (part of the buildup to the Chinese Exclusion Act). Though his advocacy was unsuccessful in staving off the Exclusion Act, he was skillful and sympathetic, and for this the Chinese emperor awarded him the Chinese consulship.[23] He was widely respected, and after suffering a fatal collapse one day on a San Francisco street, flags flew at half-mast, not only in Chinatown, but also throughout the city.[24]

Bee's outrage over the *Altonower* affair took concrete form. He penned a strong letter to the National Board of Health (NBH) (a recently formed agency involved with national quarantine, explained in chapter 2) describing the incident in detail, criticizing the lack of an organized quarantine system in San Francisco, and urging that action be taken to prevent a repetition of such a shameful calamity. To emphasize the blatant racial prejudice behind the failure to help the *Altonower*'s passengers he added, "It is with regret that I make the assertion, but every sane person resident in this City and State is fully convinced that were these 800 immigrants

Europeans this outrage would never have been tolerated, but to the contrary they would have been provided for in a very different manner, and that promptly."[25]

The NBH, realizing the seriousness of the problem, referred the letter to President Chester A. Arthur. The president asked the secretary of the treasury, Charles Folger (under whom the Marine Hospital Service [MHS] functioned) to appoint a committee to investigate, and particularly to find a suitable site for a quarantine facility.[26] Bee's impassioned letter moved the quarantine issue to the level of the federal government and marked the beginning of a quest for a federal quarantine station at San Francisco.

Quarantine issues were under debate in other ports, too. They centered around inadequate facilities, inconsistent regulations, and, in some cases, outrageous fees. The need for a national quarantine system that would impose uniform and scientifically modern procedures in all US ports was evident. The tragedy of the *Altonower* brought matters to a head at a crucial time. Frederick Bee's criticism of San Francisco's virtually nonexistent quarantine facilities and the callousness toward the Chinese passengers set forces in motion that eventually culminated in San Francisco's modern quarantine station on Angel Island.

CHAPTER TWO

The Origins of Quarantine in America

WHAT EXACTLY IS QUARANTINE, and why was it needed? A brief survey of the history of quarantine and of the American solutions to the challenges of quarantine will help to understand the procedures adopted at the station erected on Angel Island.

The origins of quarantine go back in time to periods well before ideas about germs as the cause of disease gained recognition. Properly defined, quarantine consists of practices designed to prevent certain epidemic diseases from entering a region, such as a country or a state. Initially, the methods rested on the belief that epidemic diseases were, at least in part, contagious, even though the mechanisms of contagion were obscure and not all authorities believed that diseases were directly transmissible. As far back as the ancient Greeks, vague notions such as corrupted air, telluric influences, putrefaction of waste, and religious ideas dominated medical thinking as explanations for epidemics. The direct spread from person to person, however, of some poison or vague contamination seemed to many people an equally likely explanation for epidemics.[1] Certainly, placing persons arriving from a diseased area into quarantine at a border or a port seemed logical as a practical measure that could be, and was, implemented to keep disease out. Historically, the first disease to generate quarantine measures was plague. Other maladies gradually joined the list, and by the time the San Francisco Quarantine Station was operable, the number of diseases considered quarantinable had risen to five.

Plague, also known as the Black Death and bubonic plague, exploded into Europe in the fourteenth century, unleashing an epidemic that was one of the worst in the history of humankind. Probably brought to Europe from Asia, traveling over Mongol trade routes, it slipped first into the port of Messina, Sicily, in the fall of 1347. From there it followed the commercial routes of traders and merchants throughout the Mediterranean area and Europe, spreading devastation. Estimates are that one-third to one-half of the European population perished in the wake of plague.[2] Governments and towns were terrified and erected what barriers they could.

Plague is caused by the bacterium *Yersinia pestis,* named after one of its codiscoverers, Alexandre Yersin. It is principally a disease of rats, transmitted from one rat to another by the bites of fleas. If a rodent host dies, the infected fleas, searching for another meal, may jump to a nearby human, passing on the bacteria as it feeds. From the infected flea bite, the injected germs travel to the nearest lymph glands to form inflamed, painful, pus-filled swellings called buboes (hence the word "bubonic"). Recovery is possible in that stage, but frequently the bacteria move out of the buboes and into the bloodstream, producing septicemia and usually death. If bacteria reach the lungs and are expelled during a cough, a nearby person inhaling them will almost certainly succumb to plague pneumonia, the most rapid form of death. Thus, plague epidemics can arise both through bites of infected fleas and through inhalation of coughed material.

In 1894 Alexandre Yersin and Kitasato Shibasaburo, using microscopes and laboratory cultures, both detected the organism for the first time during an outbreak in Hong Kong. Several years elapsed before scientists realized the importance of rats in plague transmission, and, while suggested as early as 1898 by a French investigator, Paul-Louis Simond, the medical community did not fully recognize the flea as the transmitter of the disease until 1906.[3] In short, when the Angel Island Quarantine Station opened in 1891, the cause and mode of transmission of plague were still obscure.

In 1377 the Dalmatian port of Ragusa, then an independent city-state and now known as Dubrovnik, Croatia, invoked the first well-documented maritime quarantine.[4] Thirty days of observation, a period called the *trentino,* became mandatory for all passengers and goods arriving by sea. The city established a sort of hospice to hold arriving detainees for the thirty days. After several adjustments, a final waiting period of forty days, the *quarantina* (the origin of the word quarantine), became the standard. Other European cities adopted similar laws.[5]

In 1423 residents of Venice coined the term "lazaretto" for the local hospice holding travelers in quarantine, a term that persisted into the twentieth century. The name stems from the Order of Saint Lazarus, an order that founded hospitals during the Crusades to care for lepers in the Holy Land. Recent excavations at the Venice lazaretto, the Lazzaretto Vecchio, located on a small island in the Venetian Lagoon, have revealed several mass graves, a testimony to plague's malignancy.[6] Lazzarettos varied in quality, and generally offered few residential comforts.[7]

Many ports also erected buildings for cargo disinfection. Following the traditional beliefs about corrupted air and putrefaction, it was common to burn coal tar pitch within ship hulls and apply a coat of vinegar to neutralize the alleged corruptions. Liberal exposure to sun and air, and sometimes seawater, was thought to purify cargo, bedding, and so forth.[8] In some ports passengers might be held on board ship for the stipulated period, in lieu of using land facilities.

To avoid unnecessary quarantines in an age when news traveled slowly, agents were often assigned to foreign ports to assess local health conditions. If the port was considered free of epidemic disease, the agent could issue a bill of health to a departing ship that would allow the vessel to avoid quarantine delays at home.[9] Reports were, unfortunately, not always accurate, but the practice continued.[10] Quarantine regulations varied from place to place, partly due to a lack of scientific knowledge, sometimes as a form of economic leverage to hinder competitors, and sometimes due to bureaucratic laxity.[11] Looking back from modern times, it is not clear how effective quarantines were, although continued outbreaks of disease suggest that they had limited success.

The next malady to invoke quarantine, yellow fever, was virtually unknown until Columbus's voyage opened up the New World to Europeans. The familiar diseases—smallpox and measles—introduced from Europe wreaked havoc among native inhabitants in the Americas, but yellow fever struck down Europeans and natives alike. The disease had existed in Africa for centuries and undoubtedly reached the Americas on slave ships sailing from Africa's west coast.[12]

Yellow fever first exploded in Barbados in 1647, where it exacted a toll of about six thousand lives. Ruinous outbreaks in Cuba and the Yucatan Peninsula followed soon after.[13] The medical profession was in the dark about the cause. A recurring theme was its apparent introduction to an area by an arriving ship, suggesting that quarantine of vessels arriving from certain designated ports was a logical way to prevent the disease from reaching shore. In faraway New England, for example, the Massachusetts Bay Colony established the first quarantine in North America, in 1647, to keep out yellow fever believed to arrive on ships from Barbados.[14]

Yellow fever is a viral disease passed to humans through the bite of a mosquito belonging to the genus *Aedes*. It was not until 1900, well after the Angel Island facility had opened, that Walter Reed and his colleagues, working in Cuba, established the mosquito as the transmitter of the virus. The course of the disease was carefully observed in the soldiers posted there during the Spanish-American War. They initially complained of fever, chills, weakness, and nausea. Next, as the virus invaded the liver, their eyes and skin turned yellow and their urine darkened. Nausea often intensified, progressing to the vomiting of blood, or "black vomit." About one-fourth to one-third of those infected died with failing livers and bleeding stomachs, while the survivors remained immune to further infection.

New Orleans, because it traded actively with Cuba and other Caribbean ports, suffered frequent yellow fever epidemics, as did other southern ports. Thus, in the New World it was primarily the fear of yellow fever that drove early quarantine measures. Ignorance of the mosquito transmission of the virus rendered the traditional measures only partially effective.

Almost two hundred years passed before the roster of epidemic diseases included a third disorder requiring quarantine: cholera. For many years it had been recognized as a localized problem in India, but matters changed in 1817 as ships and caravans plied ever-expanding trade routes, reaching more distant territories. Cholera germs accompanied the trade goods on commercial routes, spreading misery and death.[15] It was the first of several cholera pandemics.

Cholera is acquired by ingestion of food or water contaminated with the organism *Vibrio cholera*. The German scientist Robert Koch, one of the fathers of bacteriology, isolated the germ in 1884 in Egypt. The onset is sudden, starting with copious watery diarrhea, the stools so voluminous they resemble water studded with grains of rice (which are actually small pieces of sloughed-off intestinal lining). Several liters of diarrheal fluid can be lost within a few hours, rendering the sufferer weak, hypotensive, and dehydrated. Without treatment, the profound dehydration confers a mummified, greenish appearance to the face, and blood taken from a vein resembles tar. Death comes soon after. If one survives the severe diarrhea, recovery is the rule.[16]

The cholera pandemic of 1817 spared Europe, but the next pandemic did not and reached Western Europe in 1832. Although specialists argued over whether this was a contagious disease, authorities invoked quarantines.[17] Despite those precautions, cholera jumped across the Atlantic to the United States.[18] Incidentally, the epidemic occurred during a time of religious fervor in America. President Andrew Jackson was under pressure to proclaim a national day of fasting and humiliation to stem the outbreak. He indicated, in reply, that this would exceed his constitutional powers and urged church communities to recommend their own days of prayer.[19]

Following the discovery of gold in California, fortune-seekers rushing westward brought cholera to San Francisco, arriving both over land and sea routes.[20] Subsequent waves of worldwide cholera pandemics surged out of India over the next decades. The fifth pandemic, originating in 1881, swept through China and Japan, from where, once again, cholera threatened San Francisco by the sea route.[21] Fear arising from this pandemic was a factor stimulating the establishment of a quarantine station in San Francisco.

The chaos generated by cholera is what brought nations together for the first time to discuss international preventive measures, especially quarantine. The First International Sanitary Conference was convened by France in 1851.[22] Representatives of eleven European states met in Paris with good intentions, but a lack of scientific knowledge severely hampered the discussions. The deputies could not agree on whether cholera was or was not contagious, or whether quarantine was an effective barrier. After six months of deliberations, the conference was declared a success, but no international rules were established. Subsequent conferences, with cholera high on the agenda, failed to produce better results. Even at the sixth conference, in 1885, a year after Robert Koch had isolated the cholera bacillus, the members did not achieve a consensus.[23] Decisions on quarantine against cholera remained in local hands and regulations continued to vary.

Two more diseases became subject to quarantine: smallpox and typhus. Smallpox, described in chapter 1, at one time was so ubiquitous as not to be unusual. After an incubation period that can last up to nineteen days but rarely exceeds fourteen days, fever, headache, and overall malaise make an abrupt appearance. Within a few days, small pox, or fluid-containing vesicles, appear on the skin and in the mouth and throat. In severe cases these lesions coalesce, producing a sloughing of much of the skin. The mortality is high, and those who recover usually have permanent scarring of the affected skin. The virus is spread from the mouth, where lesions are present, and the skin. Fairly close contact, such as that found in a crowded passenger vessel, is optimal for dissemination. But with vaccination, a measure introduced about 1800, prevention was possible.[24] Communities thus used quarantines and vaccinations as ways to prevent further spread of the virus; San Francisco, using both techniques, was no exception.

Typhus, a louse-transmitted disease due to a tiny bacterium known as *Rickettsia prowazekii,* was the fifth of the quarantinable conditions. It is common in prisons, in wartime, and sometimes on ships. It devastated Napoleon's army during his ill-fated Russian campaign. In San Francisco, typhus rarely made an appearance and was of little concern to quarantine authorities.

In 1891, then, the year the San Francisco Quarantine Station opened on Angel Island, the mode of transmission of only one of the quarantinable diseases, cholera, was understood correctly. The understanding of transmission of smallpox, in the absence of knowing the germ, was close enough to be useful. Quarantine measures aimed at the other diseases remained empirical and were modified as scientific knowledge advanced.

In the late nineteenth century, the discoveries of Louis Pasteur in France and Robert Koch in Germany, the principal founders of the new field of bacteriology, made it clear that most so-called fevers were distinct diseases caused by specific organisms and did not arise from miasmas or putrefaction. The new knowledge opened novel ways to approach disease, as well as quarantine. The length of incubation periods of contagious diseases, their means of transmission, and methods of applying disinfection techniques to prevent the spread of germs were themes now amenable to research. The new medical knowledge also boosted nascent movements in the field of public health.

It is of singular interest that the quarantine procedures adopted at Angel Island originated in New Orleans. Quarantine was of particular urgency in New Orleans and other southern American ports, where outbreaks of yellow fever regularly menaced the population during summer months. Summer after summer, yellow fever stalked new victims in southern waterfront cities, sometimes exploding into major epidemics.[25]

Majority opinion held that yellow fever arrived by ship from the West Indies, spurring southern ports to invoke lengthy quarantines during the yellow fever season. Merchants and ship owners, fretting over the crippling effects of the resultant delays on trade, had often tried to skirt around quarantine regulations. Consequently, the new germ theories provided new hope for traders and health authorities alike. There might be a way to cleanse, or disinfect, a ship so thoroughly that, as long as there was no illness on board, it could be allowed to pass safely without a lengthy waiting period. It seemed worth a try. (Knowledge of yellow fever transmission by mosquitoes was yet to come.)

The first to describe such a technique appears to be Dr. Alfred W. Perry, professor of medical chemistry at the Charity Hospital Medical College in New Orleans and a quarantine officer at the Mississippi Quarantine Station serving New Orleans. An early advocate of the germ theory, he had already participated in spraying houses of yellow fever victims with an antiseptic, carbolic acid, to rid them of "germs."[26] The idea was easily applied to incoming ships, the presumed source of yellow fever outbreaks. Perry summarized his thoughts in a paper to the American Public Health Association in 1873, describing a cleansing technique that would not delay commerce.[27] One sentence in the paper is remarkable for its prescience: "The modern investigation of those diseases which become epidemic has continually diminished the number of those diseases which were supposed to spread by atmospheric diffusion over long distances, or which are caused by some peculiar condition of the air, and has rendered it almost certain that all epidemic diseases spread only by solid disease germs which must be carried from place to place by human intercourse."[28]

To put this statement in context, the surgeon Joseph Lister, the first to recognize bacteria as the cause of purulence in surgical wounds, published his first paper in 1867.[29] Robert Koch, the father of bacteriology, published his landmark paper on the cause of anthrax, the first incontestable demonstration of the bacterial cause of a human disease, in 1876.[30] Over the next eight years the bacteria that caused leprosy, gonorrhea, pneumonia, typhoid fever, tuberculosis, cholera, and diphtheria were isolated and studied.[31] Perry was, then, among the most forward thinkers in this field.

As a presumably foolproof disinfection method, Perry proposed to pump sulfur dioxide fumes (called by him sulfurous oxide, a potent antibacterial agent) under pressure into the holds of ships, using steam-powered air pumps installed on a tug placed alongside. In addition, disinfectants would be poured into the bilge and brushed on decks and walls, while heat or steam in a separate apparatus would sterilize clothing, bedding, and the like. Once this was completed, provided no passengers were sick, the ship could proceed.[32] Dr. Perry announced at one point that "this disinfection was more complete than has ever been performed anywhere in the world."[33] The procedure was one of cleansing, or disinfecting, possibly contaminated vessels, combined with quarantine of passengers in case of illness on board.

New Orleans implemented the procedures which, for a while, seemed to be effective, though they were accompanied by a mandatory ten-day detention period for ships from yellow fever ports. In 1876, expressing confidence that Perry's methods had reduced the yellow fever threat (and in response to business interests generally opposed to quarantines), the ten-day detention requirement was dropped. The only delay, if no one sick was on board, was for the disinfection.

Unfortunately, strict vigilance wavered. In 1878 a massive, fierce, overwhelming epidemic of yellow fever, starting in New Orleans, roared over the southern landscape, scarring the area for years to come, and changing the practice of quarantine forever. Fear gripped every neighborhood in New Orleans, sending 40,000 inhabitants fleeing for safer ground on riverboats and land routes, taking the virus with them. Upriver, Memphis suffered heavily, and other cities faced similar tragedies; for the first time, states deeper in the interior, such as Ohio, felt the wrath of a southern epidemic. The overall tally, recognizing the vagueness of the figures, was something more than 100,000 cases and up to 20,000 deaths.[34] A steamship from Havana, the *Emily B. Souder*, was the presumed source. Some of its crewmembers were ill, two died, and doctors had diagnosed their disorder incorrectly as malaria.

The terrible loss of life, the stunned economy, and the dismal reputation acquired by New Orleans aroused a combination of local and national protests. Dr. John M. Woodworth, chief of the MHS, formed a committee of experts to study the epidemic, whose deliberations achieved little.[35] In New Orleans the ten-day detention period was resumed, along with vigorous ship disinfection.[36] State funding was insufficient, though, to purchase and operate the machinery needed to maintain the Perry method correctly. Some captains, angered over the high charges, apparently steamed right through without penalty.[37]

A firm hand was needed, and it came with the accession of Dr. Joseph Holt to the presidency of the Louisiana State Board of Health in 1884. Holt, a professor of obstetrics who was interested in public health, had been an inspector for the New Orleans Department of Health.[38] More importantly, he was a persuasive man. One observer characterized his opening speech to the board of health as "more like the cant of a ward politician than what should come from the president of a board of health."[39] He recommended a rigidly enforced ship disinfection procedure and more funds.[40]

That spring, the governor, possibly prompted by Holt, announced a startling forty-day quarantine detention period for all ships from infected ports. But, argued Holt, with a government appropriation of $30,000 to improve the disinfection process, captains could avoid the forty-day detention. The reluctant legislature caved in and voted the $30,000.[41] The quarantine system that Holt established, labeled "maritime sanitation," became the model that was adopted by several states, by the MHS, and at Angel Island.

Holt's method was based on Perry's formula. During the yellow fever season, only one approach to the Mississippi River remained open. Quarantine personnel met all incoming ships to inspect the crew and passengers. After detaining in quarantine anyone suspected of harboring a contagious disease, the ship underwent cleansing. The vessels carrying no illness underwent disinfection only. Those from noninfected ports that passed inspection entered without disinfection.

The disinfection process was considered the key. The luggage and clothing of the passengers went into a large, $60 \times 11 \times 7$-foot insulated wooden container with separate compartments, drawers, and racks. Steam under pressure heated the interior to 230 degrees. Items easily damaged by steam received instead a coating of mercuric chloride.[42] To cleanse the ship, a specially outfitted tug pulled alongside, from which a large galvanized iron hose pumped sulfur dioxide fumes under pressure into the hold. Cargo usually remained in place. The hatches were closed for several hours, then opened for airing. A solution of bichloride of mercury, in a 1:500 to 1:1000 dilution, was brushed over the cabins, bilge, deck, and other surfaces. The ship might be detained up to five to seven days, depending on its point of origin.[43]

Holt, through the Louisiana State Board of Health, requested a review of the process by the MHS, whose recently established laboratory on New

York's Staten Island was capable of modern bacteriologic techniques. The MHS dispatched Dr. Joseph Kinyoun, chief of the lab, who placed culture plates in strategic spots. Although some bacteria stubbornly survived in areas buried deep in bales of material or rags, Kinyoun generally approved of the process. "The principles of the methods of disinfection are correct, but faulty in their application," and "the establishment of the present style of apparatus is a great stride in the right direction" were comments in his report.[44]

Holt increased the concentration of fumes and the exposure times and installed a new sterilizing chamber, made of steel and able to withstand higher steam pressures.[45] Word of the technique spread, and physicians from around the nation visited the New Orleans facility. John Rauch, of the Illinois State Board of Health, considered it the best system in the country, if not the world.[46] Charleston, South Carolina, adopted the system promptly, and at a quarantine conference in Montgomery, Alabama, the system was deemed the best available.[47] Dr. Wolfred Nelson, a Canadian experienced in tropical diseases, visited the facility in 1885 and reported favorably on it to the California State Board of Health three years later. He called it "an ideal quarantine."[48] Dr. John Hamilton, chief of the MHS, adopted Holt's maritime sanitation process after the MHS assumed national quarantine responsibilities in 1888.[49] The system was on exhibit at the International Medical Congress at the Chicago World Fair in 1893 and received favorable coverage in the *Journal of the American Medical Association,* an important stamp of approval.[50]

If Holt's maritime sanitation program was to become a standard for the nation, a natural choice to administer it was a federal agency. The program fit well with the new germ theory and evolving public attitudes on public health. The importance of public health had recently been highlighted by problems of sewage and waste disposal, polluted water supplies, and the like in the setting of denser urban populations. Measures to deal with these problems and enhance community health had won approval in several states.

The idea, however, that a single federal service should control quarantine in all ports of the nation ran into sharp resistance at a time when states' rights was a dominant political concept. Health (and quarantine) matters, to many states, were off-limits to central control. Additionally, quarantine duties were often a source of patronage jobs, and the fees charged provided a coveted source of revenue.[51]

A congressional act in 1799 had placed federal quarantine duties under the secretary of the Treasury but restricted them to assisting state and local authorities.[52] With some variations during the Civil War, this status held through the 1878 epidemic. Quarantine procedures remained under local or state control and, unsurprisingly, varied from port to port, a source of irritation to shipping firms. Advocates for a federal system argued for uniformity in techniques and the use of trained personnel who were not influenced by local politics. Shipping companies agreed, tired of coping with confusing regulations, substantial quarantine fees, and, in some cases, one port quarantining another as a form of economic warfare.[53]

Two contenders for a federally administered quarantine service emerged: the MHS and the NBH. The MHS was created in 1798 to provide medical care to sick and disabled seamen, and was funded through a modest deduction from their wages.[54] To remedy a period of neglect after the Civil War, in 1871 the secretary of the Treasury (under whom the MHS operated) appointed a new director, John Maynard Woodworth, to reinvigorate the MHS.[55] Woodworth, only thirty-three years old, had dark hair, keen eyes, and a generous mustache; he had been a sanitary inspector for the Chicago Department of Health. He had served as chief medical officer during William Sherman's march to the sea during the Civil War, during which, thanks to establishing strict hygienic procedures and an efficient ambulance service, he brought all of the wounded and diseased soldiers to Savannah without a single fatality.[56]

Woodworth reorganized the MHS substantially. He closed or upgraded outmoded hospitals and put the MHS's finances in the black. He created a military-style organization, complete with uniforms, ranks, and centralized administration. Furthermore, he introduced rigorous entrance examinations for medical personnel to eliminate patronage and improve quality. He awarded promotions on merit. Woodworth, firmly on the side of a national quarantine service, argued that the MHS was the most natural organization to assume this role because it already had hospitals in major ports and was familiar with the diseases of ports and sailors.[57] He advocated an approach that included uniformity in quarantine regulations, collection of health information from overseas consulates (not a practice at the time), and the use of scientific and epidemiologic information to aid in decisions.[58]

The other contender for national control of quarantine was the NBH, a body promoted by the American Public Health Association and its secretary, John Shaw Billings. The American Public Health Association was formed in 1872 as a multistate response to mounting health problems stemming from the country's rapidly growing population and crowded urban centers. Billings and the American Public Health Association, believing that the country was unprepared for a national public health body (few states even had health departments, for instance), argued for gathering more statistical data and aimed to form state health organizations as the first step. The formation of an NBH could accomplish this and standardize quarantine.[59]

The arguments ricocheted around Washington until the great yellow fever epidemic of 1878 frightened Congress into action. Congress first gave the MHS responsibility for quarantine; the following year, however, under prodding from Billings, Congress created the NBH and granted it quarantine authority. (Chinese consul Fred Bee's letter was addressed to the NBH.) The NBH, however, was still restricted to advising local quarantine services and it was funded, fatally, for only four years.[60]

Eleven days after Congress passed the NBH measure, John Woodworth died suddenly, his dream unfulfilled. His replacement, John Hamilton, also a Civil War veteran, was equally intelligent and forceful, and had already made a reputation by modernizing an MHS hospital in Boston.[61] He lobbied Congress further, pointing out that the MHS had the resources to act quickly in case of contagious disease threats while the NBH was not so equipped. As the funding for the NBH ran out, the MHS assumed a greater role in advising quarantine stations.

Congress acquiesced further in 1888 with a new quarantine law, handing additional funding to the MHS and authorizing the establishment of eight quarantine stations under MHS control. One of them was to be in San Francisco.[62] Like the NBH, the MHS could take over a local quarantine service only if requested or standards were not met; otherwise, it could only advise.[63] The NBH continued on paper until 1893, but with little authority and no funding, it expired quietly.[64]

Hamilton moved ahead. He established an interstate quarantine system, and in 1897 he opened a bacteriology laboratory in the MHS on Staten Island, New York.[65] He ambitiously named it the National Laboratory of Hygiene, and it is there that Joseph James Kinyoun tested the Holt system from New Orleans. The laboratory moved later to Washington, DC, where over time it expanded into the National Institutes of Health, one of the most renowned research institutes of the world.[66]

Uniforms, titles, and pay grades, under Hamilton, by 1889 corresponded to those of the Army and Navy.[67] Standards for the medical officers were high: One of the officers, some years later, in 1906, described the requirements for admission to the MHS to a potential applicant. The applicant's age must be between the ages of 22 and 30, he must be a graduate of a reputable medical college, must furnish two letters affirming moral and professional character, and must take three examinations: a physical examination; a general knowledge examination covering literature, language, history, geography, and general science; and finally, he must be examined in medical subjects, including anatomy, physiology, materia medica (pharmacology), internal medicine, surgery, obstetrics and gynecology, hygiene (public health), pathology, and bacteriology (the newest subject and still a mystery to many older doctors). In addition, he must show clinical proficiency by examining one or more patients and reporting on them. A grade of 80 or better out of 100 was required to pass.[68] Compared to the requirements of many medical schools of the day, when most students lacked a college degree and the medical curriculum was often skimpy, the standards were demanding and the level of officer high. Several went on to distinguished careers in public health.

Hamilton adopted the Holt method as a uniform standard, inviting local quarantine services to accept it. Before long, quarantine stations around the country were yielding their services to the MHS, with only a few holdouts. The MHS modernized or even rebuilt the stations, implementing the Holt techniques.

California closely followed the debates over control of quarantine services. San Francisco was, after all, the busiest port on the west coast, and Hamilton had already voiced the need for a proper station at the port.[69] The tragic episode of the SS *Altonower* clearly illustrated the lame status of the local quarantine services. The MHS stood ready, able to assemble a quarantine service with trained personnel and using equipment for maritime disinfection derived from Joseph Holt's original apparatus in New Orleans. The need for the facility was easier to visualize than to bring to fruition, however. Establishing a modern facility in the busiest western port, potentially threatened with cholera and smallpox, turned out to be a quarrelsome affair, one that California politicians and medical men wrestled with for years.

CHAPTER THREE

Choosing a Site

QUARANTINE ACTIVITY in San Francisco actually began during the Gold Rush, well before the shameful episode of the SS *Altonower*. The discovery of the precious metal in 1848 unleashed an extraordinary mass migration to California, drawing fortune-seekers from around the globe. Along with their meager possessions, a few travelers brought the germs of cholera, some picking up the infection in New Orleans and carrying it overland to the goldfields. Others went by sail to Panama, crossed the isthmus picking up the germs along the way, and reached San Francisco in the fall of 1850 on board the steamship *Caroline*. The pestilence tore through the city and the nearby goldfields, killing off miners and city-dwellers alike before their dreams could be realized.[1]

The state legislature responded to the epidemic by establishing a board of health in San Francisco that year and assigning it quarantine duties. The health officer was to inspect incoming vessels for evidence of communicable disease and hold them in quarantine if deemed appropriate. The legislature stipulated the construction of a building to house exposed but well passengers, but the structure never materialized.[2] The very next year the city abolished both the Quarantine Act and the San Francisco Department of Health. Cholera had disappeared and there seemed no need to continue a health department. (In fact, health departments tended to come and go in many cities in those days, for similar reasons).[3] In 1865, on reconsideration, the city resurrected a skeletal health department whose duties were primarily those of quarantine, recording vital statistics including causes of death, and promoting smallpox vaccination.[4] Within the next year the state legislature created a new San Francisco Department of Health with similar duties but specifying a separate position for a quarantine officer, appointed by the governor.[5]

As people moved west during the post–Civil War days, enlarging cities wrestled with the familiar problems of water pollution, sewage, and infectious diseases, mentioned earlier. Railroads and faster steamship travel accelerated disease spread.[6] A particularly large outbreak of small-pox in San Francisco in 1868 highlighted the problem locally.[7] To meet these challenges, medical thinkers with an eye on the future turned to a newly created specialty: first called "state medicine," and later known as "public health medicine." This specialty concerned itself with items such as birth, death, and disease statistics; clean water supplies; sewage; toxins; and quarantine. Their goal was to maintain good community health and prevent epidemics.

A notable feature of the California Gold Rush was the number of doctors who "exchanged the scalpel for the shovel" and headed westward. Of those reaching California, several had received training in leading insti-tutions and were well off financially.[8] Two of these men, who took note of disease outbreaks and other growing health problems, cooperated to promote state medicine in California. One, Henry Gibbons, Sr., was serv-ing as professor of medicine at the Philadelphia Medical College when he departed for the gold country. Soon after his arrival in San Francisco he took charge of the hastily assembled cholera hospital and later was a professor in two medical schools in the city.[9] Thomas M. Logan, edu-cated in South Carolina and Europe, arrived from New Orleans after a harrowing nine-month sea voyage around South America, and settled in Sacramento. He kept meticulous meteorology records, became professor of hygiene at the University of California, and eventually served as presi-dent of the American Medical Association.[10]

Under the encouragement of Drs. Gibbons and Logan, the California legislature created a California State Health Department in 1870, the second continuous state health department in the nation after Massachusetts.[11] Gibbons was elected president and Logan secretary. Recognizing the importance of San Francisco's port, the legislation included quarantine provisions as a health department function.

The new California State Board of Health called for a revised board of health for San Francisco. The board's health officer, elected by the local board, served also as the quarantine officer.[12] The San Francisco Board of Health could declare a foreign port infected if there was reason to believe "a contagious, infectious or pestilential disease" prevailed there.[13] This would trigger a quarantine even if all the passengers were healthy, and resulted in some unnecessary quarantines of vessels from infected ports but with no illness onboard. Typhus, smallpox, cholera, and yellow fever were listed as diseases requiring quarantine. Plague was not a threat at the time and typhus was rare.

After inspection of a vessel, the passengers, and the crew, the quarantine officer either issued a permit to dock for disembarkation (called pratique) or brought the vessel to an anchorage designated for quarantine. (The anchorage location varied. For the SS *Altonower* it was a spot three miles off of Mission Bay, a little south of the city.) The quarantine legislation authorized the quarantine officer, after boarding "any vessels bringing passengers from Asiatic ports" to "then and there, in his discretion, vaccinate each and every one of said passengers" before they went onshore.[14] If smallpox was present, everyone onboard received a vaccination, even those previously vaccinated. If a vessel was quarantined, local hospitals accepted passengers needing hospitalization, the rest remained in quarantine onboard ship (there is no mention of an onshore facility). The Quarantine Act does not refer to ship fumigation or disinfection, but these were often carried out in a makeshift way.[15]

As ship traffic and immigration increased, smallpox proved to be the major disease threat. Lacking any designated area for quarantine, passengers placed in quarantine languished in confined spaces onboard the vessels and were usually exposed to those already ill. The inability to hold people ashore frustrated the board of health and ship captains cursed the delays they incurred by lengthy quarantines. Land facilities were needed where quarantined passengers could be housed and isolated while the ship, after a cleaning, could proceed. The San Francisco Department of Health began as early as 1873 to petition the state legislature to provide funds for such facilities.[16] The requests fell on deaf ears, repeatedly, until events gradually forced a change of attitude.

In 1876, for example, a particularly aggressive smallpox epidemic jolted San Francisco. Health authorities reported 1,646 cases and estimated another 300 unreported cases (see chapter 1). Smallpox had been raging in Hong Kong, and in that year two steamers from China reached San Francisco carrying a total of twenty-seven cases between them. About a thousand passengers remained in quarantine on board their ships and several hundred received vaccinations.[17] The quarantine officer's annual report included the specific request that "a portion of one of the contiguous islands be secured and set apart for hospital purposes, so that as soon as a vessel arrives and is declared infected the officers, crew, and passengers can be immediately transferred, the vessel thoroughly cleaned and fumigated, and permitted to land and discharge cargo." [18] This constituted the first request that specified space on an island rather than a general request for land. In the same report the San Francisco health officer was convinced that the epidemic stemmed from "unscrupulous, lying and treacherous Chinamen, who have disregarded our sanitary laws, concealed and are concealing their cases of smallpox," even while admitting that other sources were possible. [19] Blaming the Chinese for health problems was, sadly, a recurring theme, and set the tone for the episode of the *Altonower*.

The request for island space also went unheeded, but the board of health kept at it. In 1879 the health officer pointed out how effective the quarantine station in New York was in warding off yellow fever. (New York at the time used two islands—one for hospitalizing sick passengers and one for quarantining well ones.) [20] He also mentioned a new risk: cholera. The disease was active in Japan, whose ports communicated directly with San Francisco. As to the expense of a facility onshore, the health officer asserted, "The cost of one such (cholera) epidemic would support an efficient quarantine for half a century." And this time the health officer specified that acreage on Angel Island, in the Bay, was potentially available if only the state would apply for it. [21]

Angel Island possessed suitable attributes for quarantine facilities. The 1.2-square-mile island in the Bay, lying about two miles north of San Francisco and separated from nearby Marin County to the north by a narrow, tide-swept channel known as Raccoon Strait, was sufficiently isolated yet easily reachable by boat. The island is moderately hilly, rising to almost eight hundred feet at the highest. The western and southern aspects, being closer to the center of the Bay, are exposed to the relatively constant and chilly winds sweeping through the Golden Gate, a contrast to the northern and eastern aspects that are more protected and warmer.

Originally used by Native Americans as a hunting ground, it was first explored by a European in 1775 when Juan Manual de Ayala, an officer in the Spanish navy, sailed into the Bay. Seeking a tranquil spot for his vessel he found an indentation on the north side of the island, sheltered from wind, and removed from the tidal current of Raccoon Strait. He anchored his modest ship, the *San Blas,* in the protected cove, since called Ayala Cove. It was Don Manual who named the island that offered him protection Isla de Los Angeles, or Angels' Island, later shortened to Angel Island. His name for another island, a barren, wind-battered island in the middle of the Bay was Isla de Los Alcatraces (Spanish for gannet, a fish-hunting bird), since anglicized to Alcatraz, renowned later for its high-security prison. Ayala and his crew sailed away after a month of sounding and mapping the Bay, leaving the island to the Native Americans.

In 1835 the diarist-turned-lawyer Richard Henry Dana spent a couple of cold December days on Angel Island gathering chopped wood, as described in his memoir, *Two Years Before the Mast*. A short time later, the island, at that time part of an independent Mexico, was awarded in a land grant to Don Antonio Maria Osio, who used it to raise cattle. But when California became a state, Osio's grant was voided and the federal government assumed ownership, alleging that the island was important for the Bay's defense. The government built no defenses, however, and squatters moved in.

When the Civil War erupted, the government, to forestall a possible attack from the sea, established an Army base, Camp Reynolds, on the western end of the island. Guns were placed and the squatters removed. The camp erected a small base hospital in Ayala Cove and renamed the area Hospital Cove. After the Civil War, the Army maintained the base, assigning it various functions. On the eastern end of Angel Island, a quarry supplied stone for fortifications on Alcatraz and for buildings in San Francisco, up until 1922.[22] The Hospital Cove area, where Ayala first landed, became the focus of attention for a quarantine station.

The California State Health Department, mindful of the smallpox epidemics in San Francisco, took up the quarantine cause and, in 1880, made its first direct request for land to the California legislature. The legislature, in turn, asked the governor to appoint a committee to study the problem and find a suitable site.[23] The governor's committee favored flat coastal land between Peninsula Point and the end of Tiburon in Marin County, facing Angel Island across Raccoon Strait. The owner of the land refused to sell, however, and a local railroad planned to extend service into the area. The old Hospital Cove on Angel Island offered less level space and the military commander on the island, Colonel Wilcox, was opposed to having a neighbor associated with contagious disease.[24] The committee reluctantly settled on land on the eastern shore of the Bay about two miles north of Point Richmond as "the best now available," though quite a distance from San Francisco.[25]

The search for a site was ongoing when the tragic events of the SS *Altonower* propelled the quarantine problem to the federal level.

Chinese consul Frederick Bee's letter, having reached President Arthur, was passed to the secretary of the Treasury (who oversaw the MHS) with a request to study the issue. The secretary formed a committee with three medical officers, one each from the Army, Navy, and the MHS. Their investigation confirmed that quarantine facilities were inadequate, adding that construction of onshore amenities had been "prevented by the lack of appropriations" from the state legislature. The committee also agreed that the land in Marin County was the best location, but unavailable.[26] Hospital Cove on Angel Island had limited level space but was otherwise acceptable. Other sites were rejected for various reasons.[27]

Surprisingly, even after the Treasury secretary committee's pointed remarks, the California legislature declined to fund a quarantine station, either due to "apathy or indifference," according to California's governor George Stoneman.[28] Matters seemed to be at an impasse.[29]

Not for long, however. A new member of the California State Board of Health proposed a way out: bypass the legislature and appeal directly to the US Congress. The idea came from Dr. R. Beverly Cole, an obstetrician-gynecologist from San Francisco. Cole was another of the well-educated physicians that had headed west during the Gold Rush. Leaving his practice in Philadelphia, he was the first San Francisco doctor to specialize in obstetrics and had developed a flourishing practice in the city. Usually spiffed out in elegant clothes, he was a local personality with great personal charm, known also for his profanity-laced oratory. He had served as dean of the medical department of the University of California and would one day be president of the American Medical Association.[30] The California State Board of Health and the governor both agreed to his proposal to approach Congress directly.[31]

In 1885 Cole traveled to Washington for a meeting of the American Medical Association. There he met with John Hamilton of the MHS, various congressional representatives, and even President Cleveland, who all gave their endorsement.[32] With this encouragement, the California State Board of Health prepared a draft bill requesting funds of up to $100,000 "to purchase grounds and erect buildings suitable for quarantine purposes at the Port of San Francisco."[33] Senator Leland Stanford, who incidentally was chair of the Committee on Epidemic Diseases, lent his support. The bill went to Congress along with a letter to the other California senator, George Hearst (father of William Randolph Hearst), asking for his assistance.[34] It passed in the House and was referred to the Senate, where it stalled. The Senate, faced with similar requests from other states, was, in fact, considering legislation with a broader scope.

The bill might still have moved at a glacial pace had not new disease threats prompted action. In 1887 another epidemic of smallpox shook Hong Kong. Simultaneously, Congress was considering a further tightening of Chinese immigration, motivating thousands more to head for California before it was too late, particularly those previously resident in the United States who might lose their right of return.[35] Inevitably, some arrived with smallpox. In all, thirty-two different ships brought to the port of San Francisco a total of forty-two cases of smallpox over the year.[36] Quarantined passengers, as before, remained bottled up on their ships or substitute vessels for a minimum of two weeks. In one instance, on the SS *Gaelic*, 1,217 passengers had to be parceled out to three ships to accommodate all in quarantine.[37] In a separate incident, the quarantine officer had to quarantine passengers having both smallpox and typhus on the same floating vessel being unable to separate the two diseases. Yet another vessel used for quarantine narrowly escaped being sent to the bottom in a storm.[38]

One case of incubating smallpox from another vessel slipped through. Eight days after the SS *City of Sydney* docked, a passenger, healthy on arrival, sickened with smallpox after disembarking. The ship's log revealed that there had been several deaths onboard the *Sydney* during her voyage. The ship's surgeon diagnosed the last one as *purpura hemorrhagica*, a form of sepsis accompanied by extensive hemorrhage into the skin. The health authorities reasonably concluded that the supposed purpura hemorrhagica victim had actually died of smallpox.[39]

A single case was all that was needed. The virus moved relentlessly through San Francisco, reaching epidemic levels in December 1887 and January 1888. The cascade of victims overwhelmed the smallpox hospital. The city erected a tent in the downtown area to care for the excess victims until an eighty-bed addition to the Pesthouse could be completed.[40] In January, as the weather grew colder, a shortage of blankets and heaters in the smallpox hospital added to the suffering, and nurses were reluctant to show up for the low pay they received.[41] Emergency vaccination centers sprang into action, some of them remaining open twenty-four hours a day, using doctors recruited from the community to assist the understaffed health department. Overall, the ad hoc services vaccinated 80,000 people (at a time when the total population of San Francisco estimated at

330,000), with up to a thousand vaccines given in one day. Unfortunately, the vaccine was defective, offering no protection.[42] The total count of victims reached 568, with 69 deaths.[43]

Smallpox was not the only threat. By January of 1887 cholera had jumped to South America and was epidemic in Asia.[44] In February of 1888 all ships from cholera-infected ports were automatically put in quarantine for two weeks.[45] An editorial in the *Pacific Medical and Surgical Journal* summarized the situation frankly: "[The state's] quarantine establishment consists of a steam-tugboat and one medical officer, now temporarily supplemented by an assistant.... No apparatus for disinfection nor accommodation for people under detention has been provided, for the law-making powers have furnished no means. In their absence, the steamship companies employ hired vessels anchored in the Bay, where the persons, sometimes numbering in the hundreds, are maintained at heavy expense."[46]

The medical establishment was not alone. San Francisco's commercial elements complained as well. Business owners fretted over the city's bad reputation and shipping companies cursed repeated delays and prodigious expenses. On March 3, 1888, representatives of city authorities, the local and state health departments, the board of trade, and the chamber of commerce all congregated in a large meeting. Upon universal agreement, an urgent plea for a federal facility was drawn up and sent, not to Sacramento but to the California representatives in Washington, providing one additional round of ammunition.[47] Senator Stanford, chair of the Committee on Epidemic Diseases, weighed in as well. The rules in Congress were suspended "by unanimous consent" to address quarantine legislation out of its normal order.[48] As the last cases of smallpox in the San Francisco epidemic faded away, the US Senate, on July 23, 1888, finally passed a quarantine bill. It was an expansion of the earlier House bill on behalf of California, now transformed into a larger project that authorized $502,500 for the establishment of several quarantine stations around the country, including one in San Diego and one in Port Townsend, Washington. Of this sum, San Francisco was to receive $103,000.[49] The president signed it into law, the same year that Congress officially transferred quarantine duties to the MHS from the expiring National Health Board.

Congress did not determine a site for the San Francisco station, however. For that, another government commission was appointed, one that included R. B. Cole. The commission ordered a survey of Hospital Cove at Angel Island and concluded that it was a satisfactory site.[50] The cove was about a quarter of a mile wide, the sandy beach was easy to dredge, and the area was guarded on each side by high hills that shielded it from the nearby Army base and kept the winds low. The relative lack of level space was annoying but not a contraindication. The secretary of the Treasury endorsed the choice, and the US Department of War (War Department) finally caved in and agreed to share the island.

In March 1889 the US Department of the Treasury (Treasury Department) officially approved Hospital Cove on Angel Island as a site for the quarantine facility and designated the MHS to operate the station.[51] In December the Treasury Department received a license for the use of ten acres in the Hospital Cove area.[52] Plans were finalized and bids solicited.[53] The San Francisco Bridge Company won the construction contract and began work in 1890.[54]

Dr. John Hamilton, surgeon general of the MHS, planned a quarantine station for San Francisco whose design and function was based on the Holt, or New Orleans, plan. The system of ship sanitation, with modifications, had already won the approval of the MHS and of Canada for general use.[55] Construction proceeded uneventfully, and on January 28, 1891, the federal government assumed control of the buildings and equipment. In 1893 the War Department granted 14.37 additional acres of land adjacent to Hospital Cove.[56]

The transfer of the buildings to the MHS in January occasioned a celebration and tour of the facilities. Mayor Sanderson, Passed Assistant Surgeon Bailhache of the MHS[57] (in charge of the San Francisco MHS Hospital and in temporary charge of the quarantine facility), Dr. R. B. Cole, Dr. Lawlor (the San Francisco quarantine officer), Col. Lyman Bridges (in charge of the construction project), John McMullin (president of the San Francisco Bridge Company, the builder) and a number of local dignitaries arrived at Hospital Cove on the city quarantine launch, the *Governor Perkins*.

After landing at a pier large enough for two steamers they inspected the three huge steel disinfecting tanks, each seven feet in interior diameter and forty feet long. Still to be built were tracks leading into them, on which carts loaded with clothing, bedding, and other items to be steam-sterilized would roll into the cylinders. Next, the group toured the lazaretto (hospital), with its two separate wards and adjacent space for a kitchen, dining area, and nurse's room. An inspection of the barracks building followed, an unadorned, basic residence for quarantined steerage passengers, with beds that could accommodate 240 people, a dining area, kitchen, and storeroom. Toilets were water closets, and sewage flowed into Raccoon Strait. A spring supplied the station's water that was pumped into elevated tanks holding 75,000 gallons. Inspection of a boathouse and washhouse (used for storage) completed the tour on level ground. Partway up the surrounding hill, the group visited the quarters for the surgeon and other personnel. The surgeon's house was 41 by 45 feet with four rooms plus a kitchen, pantry, bathroom, and basement that had a second bathroom. Each room had a fireplace for heat. Other officers lived in a duplex with three rooms each and a furnace in the basement. Attendants occupied an old house, formerly used by the Army as an isolation hospital, that needed fixing up. Finally, the tour group feasted on an elaborate luncheon in the hospital, enlivened with copious amounts of champagne and a number of speeches. The station would be ready for operation as soon as the disinfecting steam equipment and the cars running to the sterilizers were completed, in about two months.[58]

Two months later all was indeed ready, with one exception: Congress had made no appropriation for maintenance. Bedding, food, and other supplies for housing the prospective passengers were absent, and no personnel had been hired. Meanwhile, the local quarantine service continued its usual functions. That is, until the PMSS proposed an alternative plan, on a weekend that coincided with uproarious celebrations in San Francisco.

CHAPTER FOUR

Growing Pains

IN THE BREEZY DAWN of April 25, 1891, the SS *China*, a PMSS vessel originating in China, aimed its prow at the Golden Gate. Plainly visible in the
rigging was a yellow flag fluttering in the wind, an international signal
warning of contagious disease on board. While in the mid-Pacific, fever
had assailed two individuals on board, one traveling in steerage class and
one crewmember. Along with fever, they suffered severe headache and
body aches followed by the eruption of telltale pox on the skin. The
alert ship's surgeon promptly diagnosed smallpox and isolated the two
afflicted ones, while the captain raised the yellow flag. Onboard, in addition to the crew, were 44 cabin class and 116 steerage class passengers, primarily Chinese, accompanied by a cargo of tea and silks worth $800,000.
Fortunately, all passengers and crew had been vaccinated during the
voyage. This provided sufficient immunity to dampen the severity the ill-
nesses of the two sick passengers. Potential risk remained, however, if they,
or those exposed to them, disembarked into the city.

As the *China* entered the harbor, the quarantine officer, Dr. Lawler,
boarded at Meiggs' Wharf, the majestic pier that reached some two thousand feet into the harbor. He met with the *China*'s surgeon, confirmed
the diagnosis, and ordered the ship to anchor in Mission Bay, an anchorage a little south of the usual docking area, to await quarantine orders.[1]

The shipping company, the PMSS, knew that the US government had
recently constructed a new federal quarantine facility on Angel Island.
The station stood ready but remained silent and deserted for want of
personnel and supplies. The PMSS contacted Dr. Bailhache, chief of the
San Francisco MHS Hospital, asking about using the new facility, even
though it was deserted.[2] If use was permitted, the two patients with smallpox could receive care in the quarantine station hospital instead of the
ill-reputed Pesthouse, and the remaining passengers under observation
could enjoy the open air during the day and sleep in the barracks at night,
avoiding the crowded steerage conditions. Meanwhile, the *China* could

resume its schedule after a cleansing, saving the PMSS considerable time and money. Dr. Bailhache obligingly dispatched telegrams to Washington, seeking permission and funds to operate the station. The San Francisco Board of Health hovered in city hall in an emergency meeting, deciding only that the ship would have to remain in quarantine with the passengers on board unless funds arrived from Washington to operate the station.[3] Meanwhile, as everyone waited for a reply, the rest of San Francisco was embarking on celebrations at a level never seen before, oblivious to the problem lurking nearby.

San Francisco had come a long way in the preceding four decades. The growing population had pushed the city's boundaries rapidly westward. A proliferation of new housing, commercial buildings, multiple streetcar lines, and street lighting all hastened the expansion over new ground. The once scenic and empty hills near the downtown area were now topped by huge mansions belonging to newly made millionaires such as William Randolph Hearst and the Big Four of the railroad empire: Crocker, Stanford, Huntington, and Hopkins. Recently installed brightly colored cable cars, powered by steam, transported the tycoons and their guests up the same slopes that had previously exhausted horses under lighter loads and prevented building. The new wealth was also on display in the form of banks, newspapers, stores, and a building boom that included two opera houses, theaters, the ten-story *San Francisco Chronicle* building, and the majestic Palace Hotel, probably the largest in the world. The port of San Francisco was the busiest on the West Coast and was still growing.

As the city expanded, though, a curious tourist, wandering away from the expansive mansions and prosperous businesses, could easily find ill-smelling slums with defective sewerage systems south of Market Street.[4] Epidemics of diphtheria and smallpox were not unusual, tuberculosis was widespread, and the less fortunate depended as much on charity as on public services. Distinct ethnic areas dotted the city, such as the Latin Quarter, initially named for its predominantly Spanish-speaking residents but now an Italian area called North Beach, and a more rigidly restricted neighborhood, Chinatown, where almost all the city's Chinese dwelled in paltry housing.

The Chinese had been rebuffed in the goldfields but were in demand for labor. They had proved invaluable in constructing the railroads and in farming. Thousands more worked on Alaskan salmon-fishing boats and in canneries on a seasonal basis. But in the 1870s an economic depression descended on California. Workers faced unemployment and lowered wages. Competition for jobs crystallized into episodes of prejudice and violence against the Chinese, who, well outnumbered, retreated into the small (twelve to fourteen blocks), crowded, often unsanitary, enclave of Chinatown. Somehow more than 20,000 residents made do in cramped, often damp, housing (most of which was owned by Whites) with limited sanitary facilities. A steady stream of tourists gravitated to Chinatown seeking novel cuisine, store goods, clothing, and exotic shows, but few were aware of the squalor largely hidden from public view.

The artistic growth of the city had not been neglected. The famed Bohemian Club, a noted gathering place for artists and literati of the city, was underway. Bret Harte and Mark Twain had made their mark but were now memories. Oscar Wilde had paid a brief visit and Robert Louis Stevenson, long-haired and thin, had sailed for the South Seas just three years earlier, hoping to improve his health. Currently, Ambrose Bierce, a short-story writer and caustic columnist for Hearst's *Examiner,* was a literary favorite. The sensitive poet-librarian Ina Coolbrith lived across the Bay in Oakland. Frank Norris was three years away from his first published work, and Jack London was still a teenaged oyster pirate (poaching oysters) in Oakland, devouring books in the local library. The Bay Area recognized the importance of education, attested to by the presence of two medical schools and at least one university in the city, and the University of California in Berkeley.

On other fronts, the mountain wanderer and conservationist John Muir was in the process of forming the Sierra Club. Politically, reform was in the air. Progressive movements were laying siege to the boss style of politics, and boss Christopher Buckley, the blind manipulator whose machine had dominated San Francisco politics for some time, was under a grand jury investigation. In 1892, during an election for a new mayor, voters submitted secret ballots for the first time.[5]

But to return to the final weekend of April 1891, the air was festive and any troubles the city had were forgotten. Two events prompted the celebrations. First, the internationally famous actress Sarah Bernhardt was in town. Enthusiastic crowds had filled the Grand Opera House the previous night as the forty-six-year-old Bernhardt, then a grandmother, electrified audiences as she played the nineteen-year-old Joan of Arc.[6] The newspapers headlined her performances and delighted in chronicling her other activities for an enthusiastic public.[7]

The other, and principal, reason for the lavish festivities was the arrival of President Benjamin Harrison. He and his wife were approaching the end of a nine-thousand-mile journey through the United States. The five-car presidential train, complete with kitchen and dining car, lounge, berths, barbershop, smoking room, and electric lights (novel at the time), reached Oakland, across the Bay, several hours after the arrival of the SS *China*. When the president's ferry departed for San Francisco, thousands of fireworks shot into the air, triggering "a pageant of flame and light and fire."[8] A profusion of lights and lanterns installed on masts and rigging blazed from vessels that lined both sides of the ferry's course to the city, while other craft, described as "phantom ships, their sides and spars traced out in flame," dotted the harbor.[9] Illuminated tugs moved "like dancing fireflies" through the crowded waters.[10] The warship USS *Charleston*'s guns boomed out a presidential salute in a rhythm timed to the motions of a moving spotlight, adding to a cacophony of countless bells, steam whistles, and horns howling from the illuminated boats.[11] On the San Francisco shore, from the tops of Nob and Telegraph Hills, flames from huge bonfires leapt into the sky, competing with a profusion of rockets, Roman candles, and other firework displays.

At the Union Ferry Building in San Francisco, Mayor George Sanderson, Governor Henry Markham, and a committee of dignitaries welcomed the president. Accompanied by military bands and a police escort, the president rode in an open carriage past cheering crowds lined eight-deep along Market Street, illuminated by a blaze of hundreds of hastily installed electric lights. Horse-drawn police wagons kept the surging well-wishers from obstructing the procession. The constant booming of fireworks overpowered any attempts at conversation. No wonder, since the city had promised to "keep the heavens aglow."[12] The parade halted at the huge Mechanics' Pavilion at the corner of Larkin and Grove Streets, leaving "a stream of fire from the Ferry to the Pavilion," as one paper put it.[13] At the Pavilion, a massive structure capable of seating almost 11,000 people and known locally as the Madison Square Garden of the West, the president presided at a public reception for an estimated 20,000 well-wishers before he and his wife retired to their sumptuously decorated suite at the Palace Hotel.

From the anchorage at Mission Bay, the amazed passengers on the *China* gazed at the explosion of light in the San Francisco skies. One can imagine their astonishment, confined on board a disease-laden ship, as they watched the brilliant and chaotic scene while contemplating the quarantine awaiting them.

The next day, while the city rested, the PMSS representative took action. Possibly sensing that no decision would be made in Washington on a weekend, he offered to pay the expenses and to supply needed personnel to maintain the steerage passengers and the two patients at the quarantine station, acknowledging that there was no promise of reimbursement. The MHS authorities did not object to having their station operated at someone else's expense and gave Dr. Bailhache approval the next day, provided that he remained in charge.[14] The *China* moved to the newly built pier at Hospital Cove, on the north side of Angel Island.

The two smallpox victims, an officer member of the crew and a European steerage passenger, moved into the isolation hospital, or lazaretto (see chapter 2). The new barracks opened its doors to the steerage passengers, and their clothing and luggage were fed into the huge sterilizers. In the two barracks buildings, separated by a short hallway, the passengers slept on canvas cots suspended from wooden poles arranged vertically in three layers. The water closets turned out to be insufficient for the numbers using them and additional closets were placed over tidewater pending construction of new internal ones. The fecal matter was supposed to be disinfected before entering the Bay, though a report is vague on whether this was accomplished.[15] Limited hot water was available for bathing.[16] Dr. Bailhache checked the passengers daily for signs of smallpox. The cabin class passengers, as was customary at the time, were confined to the ship for forty-eight hours while their luggage underwent disinfection in the sterilizers, then were allowed to go ashore before the ship moved to Angel Island.[17] The MHS no doubt sought to avoid annoyance to "important" passengers with this policy (there was no cabin class housing on Angel Island), but soon abandoned it as inconsistent and even dangerous. Instead, they built additional, more comfortable housing, able to accommodate all classes of passenger in quarantine. The postal service fumigated the mail and the *China* departed after receiving a dose of sulfur dioxide fumes, having avoided a long quarantine delay.[18]

On Angel Island the PMSS supplied a cook, food, blankets, and other needed items, including a nurse for the two patients. The two patients, who had been previously vaccinated, recovered readily, and no new cases appeared in the barracks. Two weeks later, Bailhache allowed the passengers to move onshore for processing by immigration authorities. The trial run of Angel Island's quarantine station was a success. There was more to come.

The station was still unopened and unfunded when, a month later, on May 30, the SS *Oceanic* steamed into the Bay, flying the ominous yellow flag alerting authorities to another case of smallpox. Dr. Bailhache opened the station once more, this time accepting 293 passengers, more than the 240 the barracks could hold. A small group of Japanese were separated from the other passengers, who were mainly Chinese, and were lodged in the warehouse. Bailhache issued a statement to the press reassuring them that, even with the excess occupancy, there was food for all. A generous supply of rice was "cooked in two steam cauldrons capable of holding 250 pounds of rice at a time" and was supplemented with meat.[19] Bailhache also minimized the crowded living conditions, saying, "A happier lot of Chinese and Japanese men and women than those quarantined on Angel Island would be hard to find."[20] Simultaneously, though, he wired headquarters that more barracks space would be needed in the future if the station were to succeed. The request went unheeded.[21] The commander of the Army base next door, Col. William Shafter, who worried about smallpox straying over to his side, posted armed guards around the station and demanded that a fence be erected.[22]

Meanwhile, in Washington, a reorganization was underway that would reshape the MHS for years to come. On the first of June, one day after the *Oceanic*'s arrival, Dr. Hamilton resigned as supervising surgeon-general of the MHS, allegedly for personal reasons. Walter Wyman replaced him. Wyman had received his degree from the St. Louis Medical College in 1873, then had worked as a hospital physician and was engaged for a short time in private practice. In 1876, three years after earning his degree, he entered the MHS. He served at various quarantine stations, including those at Baltimore and New York, and in 1885 the MHS sent him to Europe where he learned the new techniques of bacteriology. He was promoted in 1888 to head the quarantine division of the MHS in Washington. Wyman was a lifelong bachelor and worked long hours. "The Service and its personnel were to him what a family usually is to a married man," wrote one author.[23] He possessed an impressive capacity for detail, wrote a thorough procedural manual, and instituted research projects. His tenure as supervising surgeon-general lasted twenty years, during which he guided the MHS through several stages to become the Public Health Service that it is today.[24]

Two weeks after Wyman settled into his new post, and after Congress had approved additional funding, the San Francisco Quarantine Station officially opened. Passed Assistant Surgeon W. P. McIntosh and his family arrived on June 15 to assume command.[25] We can only surmise what his thoughts were on arrival. The station was rustic, with no electricity or telephone. Grass, now yellowing in the summer dryness, grew everywhere. McIntosh's quarters, due to limited flat space, perched well up on the adjacent hill. With no horses or carts available, his furniture and belongings had to be carried by hand up 237 steps to reach the house. (A request for funds to purchase a horse and cart was denied.) Inside, no carpeting covered the floorboards and, though fireplaces were plentiful, the house lacked a furnace, something the new commander requested soon after arrival. The other buildings remained empty and, except for the wind, were silent. Two watery miles away to the south lay San Francisco, emerging from the morning fog. To reach it, though, McIntosh had to take a dilapidated launch to nearby Tiburon and then a ferry to San Francisco, there being no direct run to the city.[26]

As McIntosh settled in, he found that most of his initial duties were administrative. He filled positions for a cook, engineer, carpenter, attendants, and so on, and acquired blankets, mattresses, and other items for the barracks and hospital. He hired additional small launches for transportation to and from San Francisco. No refrigerator or icebox was available for storage of perishables, and lighting was by oil lamps. The water supply, from a spring, was adequate at first but soon proved insufficient.

On the station grounds, fire was a frequent hazard and broke out readily in the abundant dry grass swept by robust winds. Two weeks after McIntosh's arrival, a blaze erupted near the station, started accidentally by local picnickers. Even with help from soldiers at nearby Camp Reynolds, it took until dark to subdue the flames. Fire drills became part of the routine and goats were obtained to keep the grass low. The spring did not generate enough water pressure to wet down the roofs of the buildings, adding to the fire hazard. Fortunately, no smallpox-laden ships arrived as McIntosh fitted out the station.[27]

The quarantine activities for the Bay were divided between McIntosh of the MHS and Dr. Lawler, quarantine officer of San Francisco. The MHS did not have a boarding or a fumigation launch, and under current federal regulation the MHS could not take over the local duties unless they were specifically requested to do so. The San Francisco quarantine officer, who did possess a boarding launch, functioned as inspector of incoming ships and determined whether a quarantine was to be declared. If he called for one, the MHS would assume what might be called the island duties—hospitalizing the sick passengers, housing the well but exposed ones, and disinfecting their possessions and mail. Out on the Bay, the San Francisco quarantine officer would direct the disinfection of the ship—cleansing the decks and cabin walls with bichloride of mercury solution and fumigating the hold with chlorine gas or sulfur dioxide, as described earlier.[28] Later reports suggest that the disinfection routine was rather haphazard and did not always conform to protocol.

The division of labor between the services functioned well at first, with only occasional disagreements. Inevitably, though, as the MHS (and its budget) expanded and ships became ever larger, the delicate balance deteriorated, sliding into periods of ambiguity and conflict.

Life on Angel Island, after the initial settling in, progressed into something of a routine. McIntosh was still hiring personnel, however, when his first challenge materialized. On December 20, 1891, the SS *City of Peking* eased through the Golden Gate. The vessel, one of the first propeller-driven liners, had originated in Hong Kong and carried, along with a valuable cargo, sixty-seven passengers, several of whom were minor celebrities. Two had smallpox.[29]

The celebrity passengers, during the previous summer, had been hunting seals near the Kamchatka Peninsula when Russians seized their vessel. The Russians imprisoned the crew, claiming that the group had, in the prior year, hunted seals illegally on Russian territory. The captured Americans languished in a Vladivostok jail for about ten weeks, after which they made their way to Yokohama where they caught the *City of Peking* to California. Their plight in Russia leaked out and had become a cause célèbre in the US media. The feisty captain, a character named Alexander MacLean, was said to be a model for Wolf Larson, the ship captain in Jack London's novel *The Sea Wolf*.[30]

The *City of Peking* docked at Angel Island, remanded there by the quarantine officer. The two smallpox cases went to the lazaretto, and those caring for them on board ship went to an adjacent building for isolation and close monitoring. The others proceeded to the barracks to be vaccinated and wait out the two-week quarantine. Men and women were separated, sometimes only by a canvas partition, and as much as possible the Chinese and Japanese were separated, in line with their own preference.[31]

Within a few days, a blast of Arctic weather swept the entire Pacific Northwest. The quarantined passengers shivered under inadequate blankets in the primitive barracks that were devoid of heating. Vladivostok might have seemed warm in comparison. The purchase of a couple of stoves improved matters, but only slightly. The passengers had to remain outside during the daily fumigation of the barracks and for the daily muster and inspection. Guards from the Army base blocked the main roads. The freshwater supply was so insufficient that a tug was hired to bring in three thousand gallons twice daily. Most of the water went for the showering of passengers, cooking, cleaning, and so on. Crews had not finished installing pipes to bring in saltwater to wash out the barracks. The station remained understaffed, prompting the steamship company to supply a cook and a nurse and to agree to reimburse for the food. Thereafter it became standard policy for the steamship companies to pay a per diem to cover basic costs of the time in quarantine.

Christmas day dawned and was reasonably festive. The staff celebrated with turkey, the passengers with roast beef. The first days of 1892 ushered in another storm, with winds reaching forty miles per hour and heavy rains.[32] That ordeal lasted only three days, at which time the two-week quarantine was finally over and the passengers could pass to immigration. Surgeon McIntosh was undoubtedly touched when, after suffering through rainstorms and near-freezing temperatures, a delegation of Chinese passengers approached him to express their gratitude for his efforts on their behalf.[33]

About two weeks later, the arrival of the SS *Rio de Janeiro*, another of the newer PMSS steamers, posed a more substantial challenge. The ship, sailing from China, was scheduled to deliver 497 Chinese contract laborers to Hawaii. Before arrival in Honolulu, though, one of them broke out with smallpox. The port authorities at Honolulu, learning of the smallpox case, refused to allow anyone to land. (Hawaii was not yet a US possession.) Left with no other choice, the captain proceeded to San Francisco, flying the yellow quarantine flag.[34]

In steerage were 527 souls, far more than the 240 the station's barracks could accommodate. Given no other choice, McIntosh lodged the overflow, including a few Europeans, where he could. Some found shelter in the dining area, sleeping on the tables or on the floor. Others moved onto the outside veranda or even under the trees, exposed to the January temperatures. A disgruntled European passenger somehow smuggled a letter to the *San Francisco Chronicle* complaining of the conditions: "We Europeans sleep on the tables in the dining room while about one-half the Chinese and Japanese sleep on the floor and the remainder on the veranda and under the trees."[35] A station employee confirmed the report.[36] The Army again stationed vaccinated guards every forty feet, around the clock, at the periphery of the station to hem in wandering passengers.[37]

McIntosh endeavored fervently to relieve the suffering. He repeatedly wired Washington for permission to purchase tents. The first reply took the form of an order to hold the remaining passengers on the ship, somehow presuming that they were not exposed to smallpox. But McIntosh presumed they had been exposed, the San Francisco Board of Health wanted the passengers to remain at the station in order to fumigate the ship, and the ship's owners insisted on unloading the cargo and departing. Left on his own, McIntosh improvised. He plundered a supply of bed sacks—rectangular bags meant to be filled with straw and used as mattresses—and nailed them up as curtains to enclose as much veranda space as possible and provide partial shelter from the elements. For those who had to sleep outdoors, there was nothing but wet blankets until the chief steward offered to take the attendants lodged in one of the houses into his quarters, freeing up some space for the Chinese. Aware of the consequences of overcrowding, McIntosh intensified cleansing efforts. The now completed saltwater pipes flooded the barracks with water from the Bay and a fumigating machine pumped in sulfur dioxide two hours daily, during which time the passengers were out of doors. Rain and cold persisted, prolonging the suffering of the stranded laborers.[38]

Finally, on February first, twelve days after the first request for tents, Wyman relented and authorized the expenditure. Though hardly constituting comfort, the tents provided dry shelter for the passengers who were living under trees and on verandas. The Chinese New Year had just begun, and the weary passengers celebrated with a number of delicacies, including "several roasted and highly varnished pigs" brought over by the San Francisco Chinatown community. It was a welcome relief from island fare.[39]

Despite rapid vaccination (apparently not performed before arrival), more cases of smallpox developed. By January 30 the lazaret housed eight cases. More came in February, pushing forward the date when quarantine could be lifted. This was bitter news for the crowded, cold, passengers. Tensions and hostility rose. A fight broke out between a steward and a passenger, and Surgeon McIntosh left a terse note in his journal: "None can leave. Any caught trying will be shot first and reasoned with afterward."[40] It is not clear exactly what orders he issued or whether any of his staff were armed. Altogether twelve detainees came down with smallpox, forcing an extension of the release date to February 28th. The total quarantine period was thirty-nine days, much of it in wet and cold conditions. The contract laborers were shipped back to Hawaii, and the sick remained until well, finally departing on March 30. Just in time, as it turned out.[41]

A scant two days later, another ship emerged from the horizon bearing four more smallpox victims among its 282 passengers. Normally Dr. Lawler, the San Francisco quarantine officer, boarded first. This time, though, McIntosh boarded the vessel first, dressed in full uniform, complete with epaulets and a sword at his side (a uniform designed by Wyman), and made his inspection. Lawler arrived at the station later and made public a rift that had been brewing between them. In a newspaper reporter's presence, he quibbled that the yellow quarantine flag was not flying over the station as required when smallpox was present. The next day's newspaper printed the complaint.[42] McIntosh fumed silently but raised the yellow flag.

Unlike the previous episode, these passengers enjoyed a smoother quarantine and better weather.[43] All received vaccination and no new cases developed. The Chinese and Japanese were kept apart, with no communication permitted between them. The reasons are not entirely clear, but the two groups almost always preferred separation, in part related to dietary differences. The quarantine proceeded uneventfully until, only three days before the final day, the familiar SS *China*, once again with smallpox on board and carrying 392 steerage passengers, arrived at the station dock. This time the passengers remained on board the *China* for the three remaining days of quarantine before landing at the station.[44]

McIntosh's tour of duty was over soon after. Rotational assignments of the MHS officers were the rule. His replacement was Passed Assistant Surgeon Duncan A. Carmichael, who arrived on May 2, 1892. It may have been a result of the unusual stress on the station or a clue to a distinct personality, but Carmichael's first note reads, "The station is in bad order, the attendants insubordinate, without discipline, no night watchman on duty for weeks, and the reports and records in great confusion." He fired one hospital attendant on the same day for refusing duty.[45] Several notes during McIntosh's time suggest problems with the employees, as well as the personality conflict with Dr. Lawler.

But Carmichael had little time to make improvements. Only three days later, he received news that the SS *City of Peking* was nearing port. The ship carried a whopping 909 steerage passengers, 630 of whom were contract laborers bound for Honolulu. Once again, the Hawaiian authorities had refused landing because of smallpox. The ship's owners, the PMSS, knowing that the passenger number exceeded the station's capacity, requested permission to use a covered barge of their own to house the overflow and pay the costs. Wyman acquiesced, and the 279 passengers who were bound for San Francisco and other US cities were taken onto Angel Island and the contract laborers destined for Hawaii were housed on the barge. The PMSS supplied a cook and attendant personnel. Two Japanese stowaways also turned up and, under orders, helped the cooks prepare the hundreds of meals needed for the quarantine.

Stress on the facility mounted. The smallpox virus attacked three more victims, two at the station and one on the barge, extending the quarantine period. Then, unexpectedly, mumps broke out among the barge passengers. It cascaded through the crowd of 630 and eventually jumped across to the barracks, leaving a trail of fever and swollen salivary glands. At this point, 918 people (including crew) were under observation, a number of them with mumps, at a facility built for 240. Supplies for food, housing, and cleaning were dwindling despite the PMSS contribution. The San Francisco quarantine officer, Lawler, now on more harmonious terms with Carmichael, helped out with supplies brought on his launch, the *Governor Perkins*. Carmichael, without a horse or cart to move the supplies off the dock, was obliged to borrow them from the Army base; requests for a horse and cart had still been denied—no funds.[46]

To put an end to coping with future obstinance from Hawaii, Wyman informed the steamship companies that the San Francisco station was not to be considered an alternative quarantine facility in case of refusal by a foreign port. They would have to negotiate with ports such as Honolulu or send the ship back to the port of origin.[47] Wyman also obtained a legal opinion that landing such Chinese workers violated the Chinese Exclusion Act.[48]

Pressure mounted anyway. A telegram came from the SS *Oceanic,* still five days away on the Pacific, announcing a case of smallpox among its 576 steerage passengers, none of whom was bound for Hawaii. They were due to arrive on May 20. Carmichael replied immediately that the station was already overwhelmed and could not accommodate them. The *Oceanic's* owners, the O&O Steamship Company, countered with a request to build additional temporary barracks at their own expense. Wyman, consulted by telegraph, promptly agreed as long as the station remained in charge, and the next day a barge loaded with wooden planks and twenty-two carpenters landed at the station. With hammers in constant motion, the carpenters hastily erected two unadorned buildings. Each one housed 288 passengers with no room to spare, precisely the number called for. The beds were simple wooden cots with narrow aisles between them. Rough, uncovered redwood planks formed the walls, and on top was a roof of wooden boards without shingles or other covering. That sufficed for the moment since the rainy season had passed. Squat toilets in a separate privy took care of nature calls.[49] Just as the carpenters hammered the last nails, however, the SS *Oceanic* telegraphed, without explanation, that it was free of disease and would not stop at the quarantine station after all. Carmichael sighed in relief.[50]

The primitive barracks and the overcrowding represented conditions that, by today's standards, would raise serious objections. At the time, however, the prevalent attitude toward contract laborers and other impoverished Asians was generally unsympathetic. A comment by Carmichael in a report, voicing a common viewpoint, is pertinent: "The greater number of those held in quarantine at this station have been Chinese and Japanese immigrants, and the accommodations have largely been made for the use of this class. Good buildings with fine finish are not needed by these people, as they soon deface and disfigure them. Cheap structures of plain material are better suited for their use. There are no suitable accommodations at this station for cabin passengers."[51]

In an illustrative incident in early 1893, arriving passengers refused to turn over the keys to unlock their luggage for sterilizing. Surgeon Carmichael, unmoved, forged ahead and steamed all 319 pieces of luggage, still locked. The hot steam was hard on certain items, especially leather goods and silks, and the Chinese consul lodged a formal complaint, asking for damages of $10,000.[52] Overall, though, passengers cooperated with sterilization procedures.

The MHS purchased the barracks built by the O&O Steamship Company a couple of years later and eventually improved them. They became known as the Chinese Barracks while the original barracks took the name Japanese Barracks. A few other ships with smallpox came to the station but never again was severe overcrowding a problem. Honolulu made accommodation for ill laborers bound for Hawaii and passengers received vaccination at sea with more regularity.

Life on the island gradually improved. In September 1892 the station acquired a launch, the *George Sternberg*, named after an Army physician who was expert in microbiology and soon to be the US Army surgeon general. The launch's function was to fumigate ships by tying up to them directly, as was done in New Orleans. Until then, as mentioned, the launch that was owned by the State of California had been performing disinfections, but now the MHS planned to assume that task. The vessel was eighty feet long and equipped with a sulfur-burning furnace and fan that could pump 1,600 feet per minute of sulfur dioxide gas.[53] It was not put into use for fumigation, though, for unclear reasons (probably lack of funds), and by March 1893 the vessel's bottom was quite fouled.[54] Meanwhile, the San Francisco authorities used their launch, the *Governor Perkins*, to disinfect ships. Later in the month, bids went out for the construction of a separate hospital for noncontagious diseases in order to keep patients hospitalized with incidental ailments apart from those with smallpox.[55]

In April 1893 a case of smallpox was admitted to the lazaretto from the SS *City of New York*. After a stormy illness punctuated with intermittent delirium, the man died. Carmichael sent the *George Sternberg* to San Francisco to obtain a metal coffin, but a zinc-lined wooden coffin arrived instead. To protect the staff, the corpse, wrapped in a sheet soaked in strong mercuric chloride solution, was lowered into the coffin and a generous layer of chloride of lime applied. The coffin was sealed, and another layer of mercuric chloride-soaked sheets wrapped around it. After dark, a small crew buried the coffin in the hill above the lazaretto.[56] Later, a crematorium was installed.

In 1893 a severe financial depression plagued the country, and the MHS did not escape its effects. The launch *George Sternberg* was decommissioned, the crew laid off, and other personnel on the island reduced, as were their salaries. No night watchman patrolled the property and the station rented launches when needed.[57] Perhaps the depression affected ship travel as well, and there appears to have been little activity on the station for about a year (and no smallpox).

As the economic situation eased, improvements came as funding permitted. Prior to 1895 the Treasury Department added ten more acres to the station's grounds. Wyman authorized the construction of a structure, called a "white house," to lodge cabin class passengers because they had objected to mixing with the steerage class passengers. Newly surfaced roads and walkways reduced problems with mud in winter, and a barbed-wire fence placed around the station fulfilled a request the Army base had made years earlier.[58]

Passed Assistant Surgeon Peckham, Carmichael's successor, in his 1895 annual report, gave a full description of the station.[59] The two barracks built by the O&O Steamship Company that could hold 576 passengers supplemented the original barracks—the Japanese Barracks—that held 216 passengers, for a total capacity of 792 steerage passengers. The latter building contained a dining room, kitchen, and pantry. A hospital for noncontagious diseases supplemented the lazaretto, allowing noncontagious cases to convalesce apart from contagious cases. Two large saltwater tanks supplied seawater for flushing toilets in the barracks, a pump house pumped freshwater and saltwater to higher tanks, and a laundry provided clean clothes and bedding. A building for attendants, quarters for the steward, and separate quarters for the medical officers met the residential needs. Cabin class passengers, until more facilities were available on Angel Island, spent their quarantine time on an old Navy hulk, the USS *Omaha*, anchored nearby and fitted out with cabins designed to be more comfortable than the barracks. Several water closets had been installed on the *Omaha*. The disinfecting steamer *George Sternberg* was again ready at the dock. Near the pier were a warehouse, a boathouse, and the three large disinfecting cylinders. Close by was a Chinese kitchen, a small wood-frame building on a concrete base where specially made large boilers could steam-cook large quantities of rice and other foods. The shipping companies usually supplied a Chinese cook to prepare meals while in quarantine, as they customarily did on the ships.[60]

The station possessed no telephones or electricity. The lack of telephone service was a festering irritation, softened only partially by the availability of telegraph service at nearby Camp Reynolds. Surgeon Peckham had pointed out to Wyman that, although the luggage and belongings of the passengers were sterilized, the clothing that they wore as they passed into the barracks from the ship was not (something that Joseph Holt years ago had noticed and remedied). Wyman agreed and ordered a temporary bathhouse erected adjacent to the pier, followed later by a permanent one. It featured rooms for undressing, large showers with hot and cold water for washing, and space at the far end for donning clean jumpers and overalls while the discarded clothing was sterilized in the large steel ovens.

By this time most medical doctors recognized that organisms commonly called germs caused many of the febrile diseases, though details of how they passed from one person to another were still unclear. Fearful that the mere presence of germs on a ship posed a danger, many ships underwent disinfection simply because they had come from ports where yellow fever, smallpox, or cholera were prevalent. Steerage passengers on the suspect vessels needed disinfection also. The idea was to remove any germs brought with them from the infected port even though no one had been ill and there was no official quarantine. With the bathhouse on the pier completed, the process for passengers needing disinfection became a sort of conveyer-belt process and the surgeon's report went as follows: On the dock, all luggage was opened and spread out. Attendants separated items liable to harm from steam disinfection and targeted them for exposure to sulfur dioxide or the newer and less damaging formaldehyde gas. The remainder went to the large steam sterilizers (later modified so that they, too, used formaldehyde vapor fumigation). The waiting passengers lined up to be inspected for signs of disease, then proceeded to the bathhouse where they removed their clothes, retaining only a hat and a pair of shoes. They entered the shower room, received soap to shower with (and were inspected in more detail while nude), and passed to the next room where they were issued a clean smock and jeans to wear while their clothing underwent fumigation. They also put on the shoes and hat that they had retained. Returning to the dock, they lined up again, were counted and checked to make sure that they had nothing on their person except the issued clothing, and their own shoes and hat.[61] If deemed necessary, the hat and shoes were also dipped into carbolic acid solution. Finally, the passengers passed to the barracks with their disinfected luggage. The cook and watchmen provided by the steamship company underwent the same procedure. The medical officer mustered and inspected the passengers for disease morning and evening until released, usually in about thirty-six hours.[62]

These procedures were, of course, for steerage class passengers only. The routine for the cabin class was simpler. A directive of the year before stated, "A cursory examination of the cabin passengers, as they pass experienced (medical) officers on leaving the ship, will be sufficient."[63]

After the Great Depression passed, the personnel staffing the station grew to include the medical officer, the steward, and eight attendants. The blacksmith, who was employed to shoe the horse, also served as the engineer to maintain machinery, and acted as plumber. Another attendant ran the *Sternberg* on its errands and looked after the other craft, and a nurse took care of the sick. A carpenter repaired and improved various buildings and a new night watchman patrolled once again. Two yardmen kept busy growing vegetables, hauling coal, doing general maintenance work, cutting and burning grass and brush to avoid fires, and moving earth after mudslides to avoid damage to buildings, such as the surgeon's quarters. A cook was in place, who made use of a new chicken yard to raise birds for meat and eggs.[64]

Legislation passed in 1893 provided for stationing MHS officers in foreign ports to report on local health conditions and ensure acceptable cleanliness of ships departing for the United States. Once MHS officers were in place at key ports, they were able to issue a clean bill of health at the port of origin, allowing the omission of automatic disinfection of vessels and passengers from potentially dangerous ports, and easing work at the Quarantine Station.[65]

The growing pains were over, but life on the island would seldom be routine. A new and alarming pestilence emerged in the waning years of the century that circled the globe with amazing rapidity: plague. The plague had been making its way slowly eastward from western China, finally reaching port cities of Asia. In 1894 it exploded in Hong Kong, devastating the local population.[66] The station at Angel Island watched anxiously, aware of the frequent maritime travel between Hong Kong and San Francisco.

At the same time a prickly question, until now on the sidelines, began to move to center stage, where it generated conflict and hostility: Who was ultimately in charge of quarantine at San Francisco?

CHAPTER FIVE

Two Competing Services

THE MHS HAD ENVISIONED the implementation of a national quarantine service. It aimed to provide uniform procedures based on current science that would be applied in all US ports. In San Francisco, the quarantine activities had by law been a function of the State of California, delegated to the San Francisco Department of Health, key members of which were appointed by the governor. Thus, California law delineated what the quarantine policies were. When the federal quarantine station first settled on Angel Island, the MHS was not equipped to offer a full range of services, and out of necessity it shared the duties with the local quarantine service, through the San Francisco Board of Health. Gradually, however, Angel Island's Quarantine Station expanded its abilities and was able to assume more functions, but the California legislature never altered the local quarantine laws. The resultant ambiguity set the stage for an aggressive turf battle. The competition played out on the open waters of the Bay for all to see and often resembled scenes from a comic opera.

At first, the problems were minor. Differences of opinion about whether a ship warranted quarantine or disinfection arose between the San Francisco and MHS quarantine officers but were infrequent. The San Francisco team possessed the boarding launch, while the MHS owned the quarantine buildings and sterilization chambers, and now kept the *George Sternberg* at the dock for fumigating ships.

The State of California levied fees for quarantine services, whereas the MHS did not. The board of health reports indicate that the fees brought the San Francisco quarantine service little profit, but the quarantine officer boosted his income by charging for smallpox vaccinations, receiving a modest fee out of the quarantine charges, and by attracting patients to his private practice through name recognition.[1]

Before long businesses and shipping companies noticed that the MHS charged no fees and found that uniform quarantine procedures simplified the process from port to port. Accordingly, they began efforts to abandon the local service and rely only on the MHS crew. The San Francisco Chamber of Commerce sent a resolution to this effect to Supervising Surgeon General Walter Wyman. The California legislature also made an appeal to Wyman and even passed a bill to nullify the state's quarantine service, a bill that the governor, however, declined to sign.[2] The California Assembly later passed a joint resolution urging the senators in Washington to press the secretary of the Treasury to assume control of quarantine. The governor then reversed his vote and telegraphed the secretary of the Treasury with the same request.[3]

Wyman was quite aware of the growing dispute. He had aimed from the beginning to assume control of quarantine in San Francisco but lacked the money to do so. After the resolutions from California reached Washington, Wyman approached Congress again for extra funds. For added effect, he raised the threat of cholera, which at the time was active in China, Japan, and Hawaii, and warned that the national government might bear responsibility if the disease were introduced through an imperfect quarantine. Furthermore, he recalled an action taken in 1892 when cholera threatened New York City: the federal takeover of local quarantine surveillance. This time his appeal had the desired effect, and in September of 1895, Congress granted additional monies, for six months.[4]

It was barely enough. The most important item needed was a boarding launch, whose cost exceeded the available budget. The only vessel at hand, the *General Sternberg,* was the fumigation vessel, that was used for pumping sulfur dioxide into ships. It was not well suited for the heavy winds on the Bay and was slow, but Wyman decided it would have to do and ordered it converted into a boarding vessel. The sulfur-burning furnace was removed, the bottom scraped and painted, and a galley installed. To continue fumigations, an old Navy hulk, the *Omaha,* previously used as housing for overflow cabin class passengers in quarantine, took on the fumigation equipment. Ships needing disinfection would now tie up alongside the *Omaha,* still anchored near the station. Wyman authorized the purchase of a second, smaller, steam launch, with the fetching name *Bacillus,* to run errands and bring supplies.[5]

To convert plans into action, Wyman, in the spring of 1896, assigned Passed Assistant Surgeon Milton J. Rosenau to command the station. Rosenau had obtained his medical degree at the University of Pennsylvania Medical School and then pursued study in Europe. In 1892, shortly after he joined the MHS, a cholera epidemic spread through Europe and threatened to reach American shores. Rosenau was dispatched to Antwerp to study that disease as well as smallpox, which was also a problem there. On his return, he worked alongside Dr. Joseph Kinyoun, the brilliant investigator in charge of the MHS laboratory on Staten Island.[6] Wyman, more recently, had sent Rosenau to California to study the purity of the San Francisco water supply. He found it contaminated in areas where the runoff of surface water after rainfall was greatest, probably accounting for frequent typhoid fever in San Francisco.[7] In short, he was in California and was experienced in bacteriology.

Rosenau assumed command at Angel Island in June of 1896. Wyman instructed him explicitly, though privately, that he was to assume all quarantine functions, and that although the local officer might continue to board vessels, that officer should not be allowed to interfere in other ways.[8] Rosenau brought sufficient equipment to establish a small bacteriology laboratory on the station. Cases suspicious for cholera or plague could now be diagnosed with precision using bacteriologic culture techniques and animal inoculation. Until then the station had possessed only a microscope and sparse ancillary equipment. Assistant Surgeon Rupert Blue joined Rosenau to assist in boarding functions.[9]

The MHS now held the best cards. A boarding launch, although it was not very seaworthy, was at hand; facilities for disinfecting ships were in place; and a modern diagnostic laboratory allowed accurate diagnoses. Infected and exposed passengers could be cared for safely in the expanding land facilities. The San Francisco service boasted its own, larger, boarding launch, a less well-equipped laboratory, inadequate fumigation ability, and little else. But California laws were still on the books, and the San Francisco Board of Health intended to enforce them until repealed.

The MHS fired the first shot. Wyman sent a letter to the San Francisco Board of Health, dated June 20, 1896, stating pompously, "Heretofore the boarding and inspection of vessels arriving from foreign ports at San Francisco *has been permitted* to be continued by the local quarantine officer because of the necessary delay in the construction of the steamer, and later because of the lack of sufficient appropriation" (italics added).[10] Rosenau fired off an immediate follow-up letter asserting peremptorily, "The National Government will begin boarding and inspection of vessels entering this port from the first of next month [i.e., July 1] or soon thereafter as practicable."[11]

The San Francisco Board of Health was taken aback and reacted angrily. After a contentious meeting, the board composed a frosty reply, pointing out that the board could find no record that their service had been "permitted" by the MHS to carry out quarantine. Nor was there any language in the Quarantine Law of 1893 or any previous quarantine legislation authorizing the MHS to take over boarding and inspection. In fact, they insisted, they were simply carrying out California quarantine laws that were in force.[12] The board instructed their own quarantine officer, now Dr. W. P. Chalmers, to take up ships' papers as before and simply ignore the MHS officer.[13]

The secretary of the Treasury, Wyman's superior, presumably recognizing the fuzzy legal position he was in, backed down and allowed certificates of pratique (certification of freedom from contagious disease and permission to land; see chapter 2) from either San Francisco or MHS officers to be recognized.[14] As a result of this standoff, the board of health's quarantine officer and the MHS officer boarded incoming vessels separately, each performing an inspection and each issuing a separate certificate of pratique. If a ship attempted to dock and unload with only one pratique, the officer of the other service refused the landing until he had inspected, and vice versa.

At first a superficial air of calm prevailed, even if the affair resembled a silent film farce and annoyed the captains. For instance, as soon as the SS *Mariposa* arrived from Australia on July 2, the boarding vessels of both services were fired up as rapidly as possible (coal was the fuel) and raced at full speed to the ship. The larger and speedier *George Perkins*, carrying the local quarantine officer, Chalmers, won the race, as it usually did. Chalmers refused to hand over the papers to MHS officer Blue for his separate certifying inspection. The nonplussed captain, "in language enlivened by picturesque sea phrases," raged against Chalmers, who reluctantly handed over the papers, allowing the exasperated captain to dock the boat.[15] The MHS's *George Sternberg* was the slower of the two boats by a considerable margin, and numerous jokes about the sluggish boarding craft embarrassed the MHS officers. The next day the passengers on a ship from Panama missed out on Fourth of July festivities when Chalmers delayed the vessel after Blue had given his permission to land.[16] The week before, the captain of the *City of Everest* was equally unlucky and had to submit to two inspections, several hours apart.[17]

In the fall, the MHS tried again to exert authority. The secretary of the Treasury issued a statement to the collector of customs in San Francisco, instructing his office to allow entry only of ships given pratique by the "national quarantine officer."[18] Once again the San Francisco Department of Health erupted angrily, and once again the Treasury Department backed down and rescinded the order to customs. (The chief of the board of health, Dr. Morse, admitted that he was in favor of complete federal control, but that as long as the present laws were in effect the board would enforce them.) The shipping companies joined the fray, declaring again their eagerness to use only the MHS services. The San Francisco Chamber of Commerce agreed wholeheartedly.[19] The tension for Rosenau was probably intense. Wyman made an attempt to replace him with the well-known John Hamilton, the former MHS chief. Hamilton still worked for the MHS and was an editor of the *Journal of the American Medical Association*, but he resigned from the MHS rather than accept the assignment.[20]

The acrimony continued to drift to higher levels. In January 1897 the local quarantine officer, Chalmers, summarized his numerous grievances in a letter to the secretary of the Treasury. He emphasized that Rosenau frequently boarded ships ahead of the San Francisco officer, often made off with the only copy of the bill of health granted by the port of origin, and often gave pratique without Chalmers' consent, thus allowing others to board ships before his own inspection. In closing, he complained of a general lack of cooperation.[21]

Dr. Rosenau counterattacked, dispatching a lengthy reply with complaints of his own. He noted that Dr. Chalmers was engaged in private practice and thus was frequently delayed attending to ship inspections, on occasions so much so that the captain was forced to go onshore to find him. At times Chalmers permitted the pilot of his boarding launch to make medical inspections of passengers in his absence. At other times he signed off on pratique without inspecting the vessel, even leaving signed certificates in his office that an office clerk could dispense if needed. Finally, Rosenau observed that the San Francisco quarantine anchorage was close to shore, tempting vendors who sold train tickets, boarding house reservations, and so on, to board ships before the quarantine officer arrived. This was not only against the law, but also created a potential danger in case of contagious disease on board. Rosenau provided ample documentation of these offenses. And he reiterated that the MHS was the only entity providing full quarantine facilities, including modern ship disinfecting equipment, a bacteriology laboratory, and buildings dedicated to the care of sick patients and observation of exposed passengers.[22]

The San Francisco Board of Health, after seeing the letter, investigated Rosenau's charges and had to admit that they were largely true. The secretary of the board of health even wrote a letter requesting that pratique from the national quarantine officer be required for entry of ships to the port, "in addition to any requirements of the laws of California."[23] The San Francisco Board of Health's position was weakening, and the correspondence suggests that Dr. Chalmers was attempting to hold on to a job for which he had little time.

Wyman, in Washington, was engaged in similar disputes with California and local quarantine offices at other ports. The Quarantine Law of 1893 had strengthened the position of the MHS, but it stopped short of compelling a takeover. Wyman prodded Congress to consider legislation "requiring the National Government to assume control of all quarantines and empowering the Secretary of the Treasury to establish or purchase quarantine stations at such points as may be necessary to the National Service."[24] His confidence in the outcome was high enough to advise Rosenau, "Do not let the bickerings of the local authorities worry you. They were to be expected. The law is, I am sure, on our side, and I believe that if the matter ever goes to the courts it will be bad for the State quarantines."[25]

Newspapers fanned the flames with more stories. In April 1897 the captain of the *S G Wilder* from Honolulu, having received pratique by the MHS officer, took his passengers toward shore on a tug, only to be intercepted halfway by Chalmers who ordered that they return to the ship or be fined. They returned, forced to tolerate a full reinspection of passengers and cargo.[26] On yet another occasion Rosenau sent several Japanese steerage passengers to Angel Island for disinfection without consulting Chalmers, giving rise to more newspaper headlines and more meetings of the San Francisco Department of Health.[27]

Wyman, mentioning the admitted failure of the local quarantine officer to act properly, appealed again to his superior, this time the newly appointed Treasury secretary, Lyman Gage, asking him to invoke the empowering phrase from the Quarantine Act of 1893. Wyman quoted from the Act, "If the State or municipal authorities shall fail or refuse to enforce said rules and regulations, the President shall execute and enforce the same, and adopt such measures as in his judgment shall be necessary to prevent the introduction or spread of such diseases, and may detail or appoint officers for that purpose."[28]

Treasury Secretary Gage and President McKinley were persuaded to act. On May 18, 1897, the president signed an order drawn up by Wyman designating Passed Assistant Surgeon Rosenau as sole quarantine officer for the port of San Francisco.[29] The presidential order listed three reasons for the order: repeated violation of both local and federal quarantine laws, no provision by local authorities for basic services (disinfection of vessels, isolation of sick individuals, detention of those exposed), and requests from the state legislature and local chamber of commerce for the MHS to assume services. Also cited was the willingness of the San Francisco Department of Health to turn over the duties, pending change of existing California laws. Wyman gives added emphasis in his annual report, writing that the appointment of Rosenau as the sole quarantine officer "appears to be an absolute necessity in order to protect the country from the introduction of foreign pestilence."[30]

At that time, Chalmers was insisting that all mail be disinfected, while the MHS had decided that that was no longer necessary. The postmaster general, caught in the middle, asked for guidance and Wyman, in his reply, invoked the presidential order, adding, "Therefore the Postmaster at San Francisco should be instructed to ignore the request of the State and local authorities."[31]

Deficiencies there may have been, but the San Francisco Department of Health stood its ground, arguing that the old California quarantine laws were still on the books and had to be enforced. The California legislature, inexplicably, failed to act; to break the deadlock the San Francisco Department of Health decided to bring the issue to the courts, where it thought it had a chance. They sought a test case.

On September 11, 1897, Rupert Blue, the MHS officer assisting Rosenau, boarded the SS *Gaelic* and granted pratique. As the ship headed for the dock, Dr. Chalmers arrived, demanding to board for inspection. The captain intentionally ignored Chalmers and pushed on. The captain and the pilot who helped dock the ship were duly arrested and charged with violation of section 3105 of the political code by preventing the San Francisco quarantine officer from making his obligatory examination.[32]

The case went to court. It attracted attention since the outcome potentially affected other quarantine stations still under local control. The shipping companies backed the *Gaelic*, prepared to pay any fine due, and the

US attorney general instructed the US attorney at San Francisco to aid and advise the MHS officers in the pending litigation.[33] The opposing forces were lining up.

The captain and pilot lost the case and were duly fined $10. The decision was promptly appealed to the city and county superior court, where the judgment was reversed. The opinion of that court noted that since California service did not fully carry out the quarantine laws and the president had appointed an officer specifically to remedy this problem, the authority of the federal officer prevailed.[34] The case was then appealed to the California State Supreme Court, but there it met delay.[35] On the waterfront, meanwhile, the bickering continued as the local quarantine officer clung to his waning authority. Meanwhile, Wyman assigned Rosenau to Cuba, replacing him, after a short interval, with the director of the MHS laboratory, Joseph J. Kinyoun. Kinyoun was one of the best-informed scientists of the country, particularly in bacteriology. He had studied twice in Europe, had some knowledge of plague bacilli, and was professor of pathology and bacteriology at Georgetown University Medical School. His colleagues in Washington, hearing of his transfer to lonely Angel Island, reacted with some disappointment. As a gesture of their admiration for his work, they feted him with a dinner in his honor and emphasized that the success of the laboratory was due to his efforts, possibly a criticism of Wyman for the transfer.[36]

Shortly after Kinyoun's arrival, the curious case of the *Nippon Maru* brought the local conflict to new heights. Japanese immigration had been increasing in recent years and Japanese ships now competed in the Hong Kong–Japan–San Francisco run. The SS *Nippon Maru* left Hong Kong on May 21, 1899, passing through Nagasaki and Honolulu. By the time it reached Hawaii, two passengers had died of plague, the second case confirmed bacteriologically.[37] In Honolulu (Hawaii was by then a US possession), the victim was ordered cremated, the passengers held in quarantine for a week, and the ship cleansed. The *Nippon Maru* resumed its voyage, buried at sea another passenger who died of what was thought to be a stroke, and arrived at San Francisco on the morning of June 27.[38] Dr. Kinyoun boarded the vessel, inspected it, and found it to be clean and the passengers healthy. However, knowing that plague cases had been on board, and under orders from Wyman to disinfect the baggage of all passengers arriving from China, he brought the ship to the quarantine station. Dr. Chalmers arrived to inspect the passengers but was denied permission to board, which infuriated him. This episode and subsequent encounters suggest a truculent aspect of Kinyoun's demeanor that would prove troublesome in the future.

Later that day, during a second inspection of the ship, Kinyoun was amazed to discover eleven stowaways. They had been hiding in coal bins and had survived through surreptitious feedings by sympathetic crew-members. The next afternoon, when all the passengers debarked at the station, two of the stowaways were missing. That same morning an Italian crab fisherman discovered two bodies floating near the entrance to the Bay. They appeared to be Asian and they wore *Nippon Maru* life preservers. Although no one admitted knowing how they escaped, it was presumed that they had been secretly let over the side of the ship during the night by sympathetic crewmembers.

At the autopsy table in San Francisco, the coroner thought that one victim showed mild swelling of lymph glands, and he took samples for culture. He determined the cause of death to be drowning, and the corpses were cremated. Dr. Chalmers and another member of the San Francisco Board of Health, Dr. Coffey, went to Angel Island to examine the quarantined passengers and again Kinyoun refused permission to land. Angered and frustrated, the board of health members voiced their outrage publicly. Coffey threatened to put Kinyoun in the Pesthouse if he ever came to San Francisco.[39]

The next day the city bacteriologist, Dr. Barbat, viewed the cultures from the drowned man's lymph glands and announced that they were plague bacilli. The board of health met in a stormy session. The members resolved that the *Nippon Maru* should not be allowed to remain at the dock (it had docked after being disinfected by the MHS and supplied with a fresh crew) and that anyone from Angel Island trying to come onshore would be arrested. They ordered the ship and its crew towed about a mile from shore. The next day, July 1, happened to be the first day that a new San Francisco quarantine officer, Dr. Cohn, was on duty. He ordered the ship disinfected all over again, much to the captain's annoyance.[40] Probably because of the primitive cleansing equipment, the ship reeked of disinfectant, mattresses were soaked, and woodwork had been damaged (although cockroaches survived). Finally, Dr. Cohn reaffirmed that anyone coming onshore from Angel Island would be arrested and placed in the Pesthouse.[41]

Kinyoun, who knew his bacteriology, soon heard about the finding of plague bacilli by the city laboratory. He was highly skeptical. He had reliable reports that the two drowned men had felt well and eaten a large meal shortly before escaping. He also believed that the bacteria could not be identified in such a short time, especially since the San Francisco laboratory lacked facilities for animal inoculation, a necessary step for diagnosis. Because of the importance of the findings and the hostility between the federal and local authorities, Dr. Gassaway, from the San Francisco MHS Hospital, located at the Presidio, the principal military base in the area, and not part of the quarantine service, served as a tactful mediator and arranged a conference.

Gassaway brought both Dr. Coffey and Dr. Barbat to Angel Island. After a venting of feelings on both sides, Barbat handed the slides over, admitting that he had destroyed the cultures, allegedly because it was dangerous to keep them. Kinyoun examined the slides microscopically and asserted that the bacteria were not those of plague, but rather a type of *Streptococcus,* an organism that causes skin, throat, and lung infections.[42] It was too late for animal inoculation. On hearing Kinyoun's opinion, Drs. Coffey and Barbat announced that they had actually presented Kinyoun with slides of real plague bacilli obtained from an outside source, from Dr. Kitasato himself (one of the discoverers of the plague bacillus), in order to test his ability to identify them. Kinyoun's diagnosis of *Streptococci,* therefore, they gloated, was proof of his incompetence.[43]

The claim that the purported plague bacilli came from another source was almost certainly false. Gassaway affirmed that he was told by other (unnamed) doctors that the bacteria had indeed come from the cases pulled out of the Bay.[44] Rancor and resentment appeared to have driven the board of health men to deceit. Furthermore, the correspondence suggests a lack of tact and restraint by both Kinyoun and board of health members. The newspapers picked up the quarrel, the *San Francisco Examiner* criticizing the federal authorities and the *San Francisco Chronicle* being more supportive.[45]

Interestingly enough, no one thought to examine a rat from the ship. The role of rats in plague dissemination was still not clear, though in Hawaii the passengers of the *Nippon Maru* were held in quarantine on a chartered ship that was subjected to rat precautions as part of the anti-plague measures Honolulu had adopted.[46]

The heavy air of hostility hovered for a few months. Competition to board incoming vessels became so heated that Dr. Coffey of the board of health threatened that he would "come on board any and all vessels as he saw fit" even if it required "a company of militia to put him on board."[47] Kinyoun responded by requesting that the Treasury Department detail customs inspectors to accompany him as he boarded ships to prevent premature boarding by the San Francisco quarantine officer.[48] The maneuver was successful, essentially shutting out the local quarantine officers.[49] The new quarantine officer, Dr. Cohn, once raced out at 4:00 a.m. to be the first to board the incoming SS *Doric* but found that US Customs officials had beaten him to it. When they refused to allow him to board, he sought out the chief of police for help but the chief wisely declined to interfere.[50]

The board of health continued to fume and sought another test case.[51] But no additional suit ever materialized. In fact, the owner of a sailing vessel, the *R. P. Rithet*, sued the San Francisco quarantine service over improper fees. The MHS quarantine officer had inspected the craft and granted pratique, whereupon the San Francisco officer gave another pratique, without inspection, and charged the customary fee. The *Rithet*'s owner protested the fee, claiming that no inspection had been performed. The court upheld his claim, saying, "As the fee charged can only be justified upon the theory of a compensation for services rendered, it cannot be recovered when there has been no service."[52]

How was the standoff resolved? It never was; it simply died out. Local politics played a role. A reformist spirit had been sweeping through San Francisco in the previous few years. James Phelan, a primary figure in the reform movement, was elected mayor in 1896, taking over from Adolph Sutro in 1897. Under his sponsorship, a new city charter, the first new one since 1856, went into effect in January 1900. It was a document designed to (hopefully) reduce the patronage and corruption prevalent in city politics. With the new charter came a new board of health. When the new members assumed office on January 9, they found that the previous year's funds, intended to last until June 30, had not only been spent but in fact had been overspent. The city reluctantly granted a meager supplement to keep the board of health alive, which sufficed only because many board members served without pay during the interim.[53] The new board of health, looking over its financial straits, the recent court cases, and the prevailing popular opinion, simply did not appoint a new quarantine officer.[54] The quarantine dispute was over. The MHS was now in control.

The period of tranquility was doomed to be of short duration, however. In only a few weeks the worst fear of both the board of health and the MHS came to pass: plague arrived in San Francisco. The ensuing struggle between Joseph Kinyoun, chief of the quarantine station, and the California authorities was monumental and unprecedented.

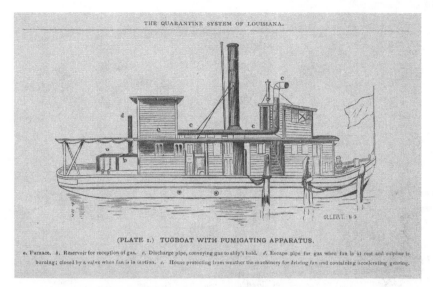

(PLATE 1.) TUGBOAT WITH FUMIGATING APPARATUS.

a. Furnace. *b*. Reservoir for reception of gas. *c*. Discharge pipe, conveying gas to ship's hold. *d*. Escape pipe for gas when fan is at rest and sulphur is burning; closed by a valve when fan is in motion. *e*. House protecting from weather the machinery for driving fan and containing accelerating gearing.

Joseph Holt's design for fumigation tug, New Orleans. From Joseph Holt, *The Quarantine System of Louisiana: Methods of Disinfection Practised* (New Orleans: L. Graham & Son, 1887). From Open Collections Program at Harvard University. Courtesy of the Francis A, Countway Library of Medicine, Harvard University. Record ID: 990056858080203941.

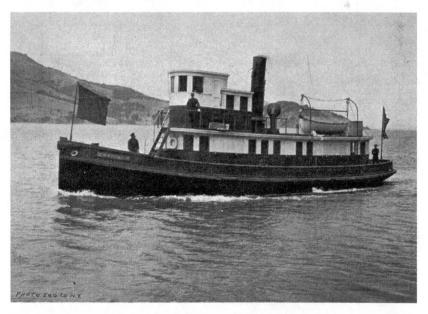

The *George Sternberg*. Used as fumigation vessel, then as boarding vessel. Courtesy Images from the History of Medicine, US National Library of Medicine. Image ID: A024257.

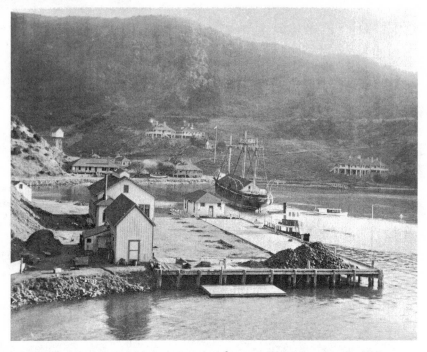

Angel Island Quarantine Station, 1895, view from southeast showing the hulk *Omaha*, used as quarantine space and fumigation vessel. Courtesy San Francisco Maritime National Historical Park. Photo number (B12.14218n).

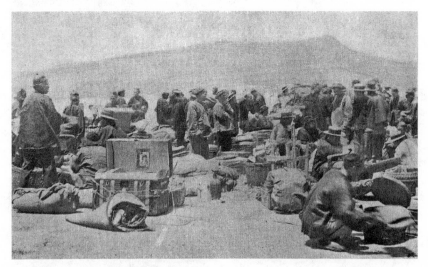

Immigrants on the Angel Island Quarantine Station dock opening baggage for disinfection. Courtesy Golden Gate National Recreation Area, Park Archives, Interpretation Negative Collection, GOGA-2316.

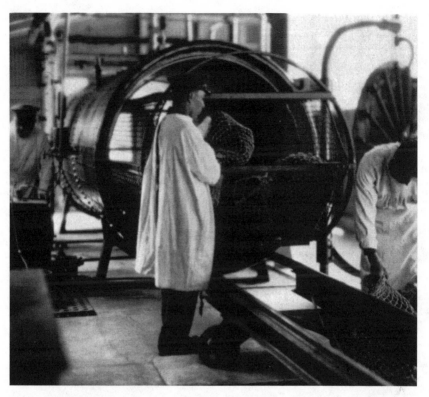

Loading clothes into sterilization chamber. The photograph was taken at the Angel Island Immigration Station but the chambers at the Quarantine Station were similar. Courtesy, Images from the History of Medicine US National Library of Medicine. Image ID: A018037.

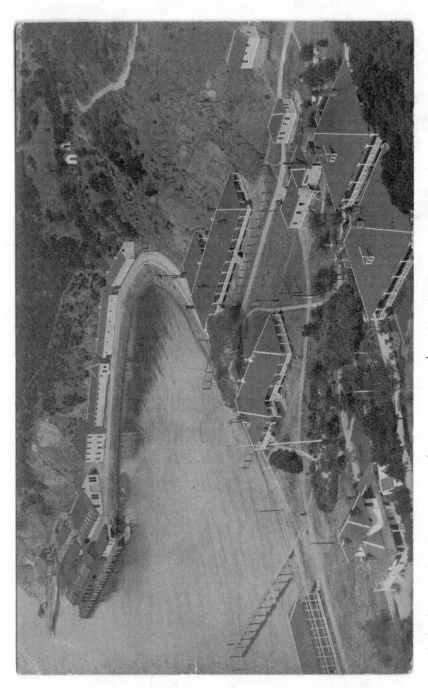

Angel Island Quarantine Station, 1911, view from the west. Courtesy of California History Room, California State Library, Sacramento, California. Image ID: 2014-4522.

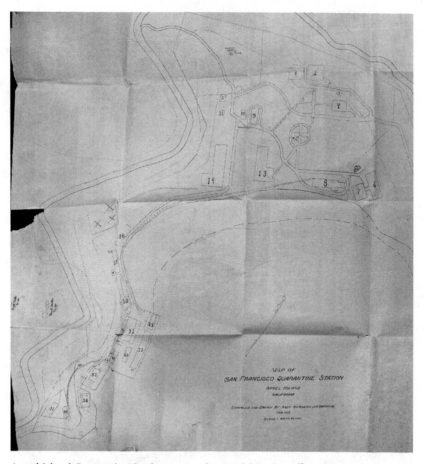

Angel Island Quarantine Station as seen in 1913. [1] Junior officer's quarters.
[2] Quarters of medical officer in charge. [3] Green house and tool room.
[4] Pharmacist's quarters. [5] White house. [6] Upper lazaretto. [7] Lower
lazaretto. [8] Cabin passenger barracks. [9] Attendants' kitchen and dining room.
[10] Paint shop and storeroom. [11] Quarters for cook and waiter. [12] Pump
house. [13] Executive building and second-class barracks. [14] Japanese Barracks.
[15] Laboratory. [18] and [19] Chinese Barracks. [20] Attendants' quarters and cabin
passenger bath house. [21] Disinfecting house. [22] Wharf shed. [23] Steerage-
class bath house. [24] Boat house. [25] Machine and carpenter shops. [26] Stable.
[28] Power house. [29] Chinese kitchen and dining room. [30] Smallpox hospital.
[31] Smallpox quarters (for people exposed but not ill). [36] Clothes room.
[37] Laundry. [39] Chinese kitchen and junk room. [40] Wagon shed. [42] Privy
for Chinese Barracks. [43] Privy for men on wharf. [44] Privy for women on wharf.
[45] Blacksmith's shop and tool shed. Courtesy of NARA, College Park, RG 90,
folder no. 3, 05119/0315. Photograph of map by author.

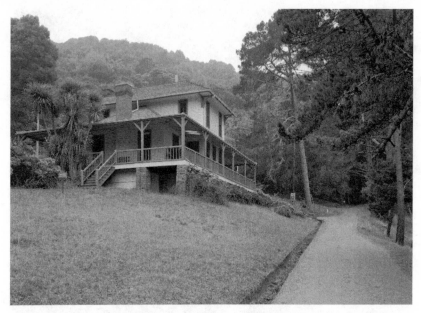

Pharmacist's house, Angel Island Quarantine Station, 1933 or later. Courtesy Historic American Building Survey, Prints and Photographs Division, Library of Congress (HABS CA-2779-B).

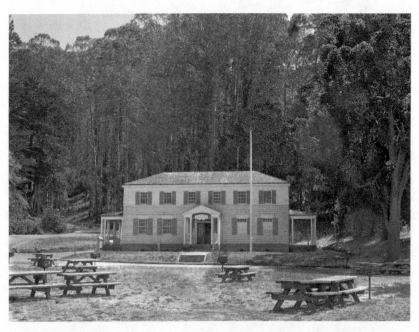

Former Officers' Quarters, Angel Island Quarantine Station, Angel Island State Park. It is now a small museum. Photograph by James W. Rosenthal, 2002. Courtesy Historic American Building Survey, Prints and Photographs Division, Library of Congress (HABS CA-2779-A).

CHAPTER SIX

Plague in the City

Knowledge slowly builds up what ignorance in an hour pulls down.
— George Eliot

ON MARCH 6, 1900, a forty-one-year-old Chinese lumber salesman, Wong Chut King,[1] was found dead in a small basement cubicle of the Globe Hotel, a once-fashionable but now cheap lodging house on Dupont Street in San Francisco's Chinatown.[2] The assistant health officer for San Francisco examined the corpse and noticed swollen, inflamed lymph glands in the right groin, a sign of an infectious process. A bacteriologist new to the San Francisco Department of Health, Wilfred Kellogg, removed tissue from a gland and examined it microscopically. Through the lens he saw stained, stumpy bacterial rods suspiciously resembling those of plague bacilli and promptly cultured them. Dr. Kellogg, who had replaced Dr. Barbat at a change of administration and had received training in bacteriology at the University of California and in Europe, had reason to be suspicious. He was aware of a few cases of possible plague that had turned up in San Francisco during the previous year and a half, though they were never diagnosed as such.[3] Mindful of this and of the embarrassing comedy over the *Nippon Maru,* he took samples to Dr. Kinyoun on Angel Island for study in animals.[4]

Kinyoun agreed that the bacteria resembled those of plague. He recultured the organisms and inoculated them into guinea pigs, a rat, and a monkey. The animals eventually succumbed, making the diagnosis of plague indisputable. But the guinea pigs and rat took eighty-two hours to die and the monkey lasted two more weeks before succumbing, intervals that created uncertainty and conflict.

The new San Francisco Board of Health, aware of Dr. Kinyoun's tentative opinion, was sufficiently convinced of the diagnosis that, without waiting for the results of the animal inoculations, declared the presence of plague. They ordered the clothes and bedding of Wong Chut King to be burned and his body cremated, and prescribed a liberal application of sulfur fumes and chemicals to cleanse the Globe Hotel. On the board of health 's directive, the authorities promptly cordoned off the roughly fourteen-square-block area of Chinatown and declared a quarantine. Ropes enclosed the sector and police patrolled the boundaries. Excluded from the quarantine were non-Chinese establishments on the perimeter, even if they were within the boundary. Exit was almost impossible. The Chinese understandably saw themselves as victims of the anti-Chinese discrimination pervasive in San Francisco. Lost wages and difficulties obtaining food became urgent problems. Those outside the barrier complained of a sudden shortage of maids, cooks, launderers, and other neglected but sorely needed workers.[5]

The San Francisco Department of Health performed house-to-house inspections in Chinatown looking for additional cases, poking through the dimly lit, meager dwellings. The Globe Hotel harbored no additional cases and none turned up in apartment searches, though hiding the sick and the dead from strangers in the charged atmosphere was suspected to be a common practice among the Chinese.[6]

The media reaction to the plague scare was one of almost complete denial. A bizarre reaction, perhaps, since the local press had recently reported the reappearance of plague in Honolulu, only a boat ride away from San Francisco, without questioning the diagnosis.[7] Newspapers, except for the *San Francisco Examiner*, ridiculed the idea of plague in their midst and cast repeated slurs on the San Francisco Department of Health and its members.[8] The *San Francisco Chronicle* referred to the news as the "curse of the bubonic plague fake"[9] and the "plague fake of the bubonic Board of Health."[10] Business interests, fearing that news of a plague epidemic would shut down commerce, also insisted that there was nothing to worry about.

Three days after the isolation of Chinatown, all attention focused on the animals inoculated to confirm the diagnosis of plague. Surprisingly, they stubbornly remained healthy, causing many, including medical men, to doubt the diagnosis. The board of health, under intense pressure from the Chinese community and business interests, was compelled to lift the quarantine barriers around Chinatown.

But the guinea pigs finally sickened and died almost immediately after the quarantine was lifted. They showed typical findings of plague at autopsy: swollen, inflamed lymph glands teeming with plague bacteria. Additional house searches in Chinatown disclosed a second case. Kinyoun was alarmed and informed his chief, Wyman, who authorized Kinyoun to vaccinate as many people in Chinatown as possible. Wyman sent out about two thousand doses of a plague vaccine known as the Haffkine vaccine, with more to follow, and about three hundred doses of an antiserum.[11]

The vaccine was named after Dr. Mordecai Haffkine, a Russian-born bacteriologist working in India and already known for creating a vaccine against cholera. Plague had decimated India in the previous few years and Haffkine had developed a vaccine against it that was considered fairly effective. Plague had erupted in numerous countries, and to meet the demand for vaccine, Haffkine's laboratory had manufactured more than 2 million doses in the first four and a half years of operation to try and fill orders from around the world.[12] The vaccine tended to cause severe reactions, leading to resistance to its use in India and later in Hawaii.[13] Only later did doubts arise about its effectiveness, though no properly controlled studies ever settled the matter.[14]

The antiserum, intended primarily as a treatment agent in cases of active plague, was a product developed by Alexandre Yersin, the co-discoverer of the plague organism, and was manufactured at the Pasteur Institute in Paris.[15] It consisted of serum from animals immunized against plague. It was believed to be effective as long as the disease was not too far advanced. Some in San Francisco also took it as a prophylactic agent, though the duration of protection was short. The risk of using antiserum was the possibility of serum sickness, a sometimes serious allergic reaction against foreign proteins in the body.

As March rolled along no new plague cases came to light. House-to-house inspections ceased on the March 28, with the hope that the infection was dying out. But it was wishful thinking. Five more Chinese fell ill between late April and late May, forcing Kinyoun to conclude that the disease was entering an epidemic stage.[16]

The San Francisco Board of Health also recognized the gravity of the problem and moved to find hidden cases and improve sanitation in Chinatown. Living conditions in Chinatown were dismal, with families crammed into tiny rooms that were poorly lit, almost devoid of ventilation, and sometimes lacking windows. Basement apartments exuded dampness and often foul odors, related to defective sewage removal.

A maze of underground tunnels connected apartments, undoubtedly a factor in hiding sick or deceased dwellers.[17]

The board fumigated with sulfur dioxide where it could and sloshed disinfectant solutions in sewerage lines, basements, and apartments. Garbage was burned. Actions were limited, though, because the city authorities, with their heads deep in the sand, refused to provide adequate funds for the work. The press even accused the board of health of milking the public treasury for its own benefit (in fact, members still served without pay, the previous board having overspent their budget.)[18]

The board of health ordered autopsies in cases where the cause of death was not well established. But the Chinese bitterly opposed autopsies, believing that cutting the body violated conceptions of filial piety, was offensive to ancestors, and interfered with the journey of the soul after life.[19] Medical authorities were convinced that frightened Chinese residents hid their sick and dead, avoiding the prying inspectors by moving bodies from place to place through subterranean tunnels or smuggling them out of the area to receive clandestine burials.[20]

Wyman, Kinyoun, and the board of health decided to go ahead with widespread vaccination of Chinatown residents, using the Haffkine vaccine. The Chinese resisted, though, and the attempt met with little success. Rumors circulated that the vaccine was dangerous and a reporter for the *San Francisco Examiner* who took the vaccine described a severe reaction.[21] The Chinese consul and the Chinese Six Companies[22] attempted to cooperate with the vaccine program but when officers of the Chinese Six Companies were asked by suspicious residents to take it themselves, they refused. "Immediately thereafter there occurred almost a riot" and some officers were "besieged in their houses."[23] Vehement protests erupted in the Chinese press. Street demonstrations followed, during which angry protesters threw stones at the Chinese consulate.[24] To smooth the waters, Kinyoun advised in May that the vaccinations be made voluntary.[25] Wyman, trying to be reassuring about side effects, stated that many doses had been given in Honolulu without difficulties.[26] But the reports of severe side effects carried more weight with the public.

Wyman, made aware that some Chinese were fleeing the city, feared the specter of further spread of plague. He drafted a report to President McKinley reminding him of a quarantine law of 1890 allowing the president to take measures to prevent the spread of certain epidemic diseases across state borders. The president assented and authorized the secretary of

the Treasury to take such measures. They included restriction of the movement of those suspected of carrying plague, both out of San Francisco and
across state lines.[27]

Regulations were issued on May 22 that restricted travel "by common
carrier to Asiatics or other races particularly liable to the disease."[28]
Kinyoun assigned agents to various points along California's borders and
on internal rail lines to prevent Asians and others suspected of plague
from using the lines. He enlisted help from the Navy and the Customs
Bureau (they had a revenue cutter) to patrol the waters around the Bay.[29]

The Chinese and the business communities fought back. A class-
action lawsuit against members of the San Francisco Board of Health
and Kinyoun was brought on behalf of a Chinese man who claimed that
requiring vaccinations for only Asians in order to travel was illegal discrimination. On May 28 the judge agreed with the plaintiff. His opinion
noted that the order included all Asians regardless of place of residence or
history of exposure. He added that the San Francisco Board of Supervisors
had never even stated that plague existed in the city and, finally, since the
number of reputed cases was small, there was no compelling evidence of
an emergency. The judge declined to hear any scientific evidence on the
existence of plague.[30]

The California State Board of Health, at this juncture, stepped in to
decree a second quarantine if the San Francisco Board of Supervisors
did not publicly recognize the plague outbreak. The supervisors caved in
and, formally recognizing the existence of plague, created the necessary
legislation to permit the quarantine and cleansing of Chinatown. Barbed
wire went up and an ample number of police officers arrived to enforce
the revised quarantine. The Chinese again found themselves surrounded,
unable to leave Chinatown. They faced shortages of food and supplies, as
well as unemployment.

The Chinatown community still resisted. Homes would not open
their doors to inspection and businesses were suddenly closed. Hardly
anyone reported sickness, and no one reported deaths. Various civic
groups tried to help but response was limited. Incidentally, it was a census
year, and census takers could enter Chinatown only after receiving the
Haffkine vaccine or the Yersin antiserum. Their interpreters were already
inside, unable to get out.[31]

Another lawsuit was filed, claiming that placing a Chinese American–
owned business under quarantine while a European American–owned

business next door was exempted was discrimination. Once again, the court agreed with the plaintiff. The areas cordoned off clearly exempted non-Chinese businesses that were adjacent to Chinese ones in the quarantined area. California governor Henry Gage himself testified at the trial, claiming that there was no plague in San Francisco. The court declined again to hear medical evidence. The quarantine was lifted.[32]

Kinyoun's response to the judgment was abrupt. To stem the flow of people leaving San Francisco he strengthened the travel ban, ordering railroad and steamship companies not to sell tickets to anyone not possessing a health certificate signed by him; in addition, he wrote letters to health boards of several states warning them about the possibility of plague carried by rail passengers and freight. In a letter to Senator F. M. Cockrell, a friend, and to Dr. Bailhache at the MHS Hospital in San Francisco, Kinyoun indicates that these actions were on prior orders from Wyman that had not been revised.[33] Meanwhile, merchants in San Francisco, beginning to see the dangers more clearly, had gathered $30,000 to aid the San Francisco Board of Health in cleanup activities.[34]

Newspapers continued to howl against plague measures. The governor fumed, and his vehement objections reached President McKinley, who changed his mind and canceled the ban on travel within California, though the MHS could still enforce inspections at state borders. As a final blow, Kinyoun's action strengthening the travel ban earned him a charge of contempt of court.[35]

Kinyoun was exhausted. He believed that he was dealing with a growing epidemic that could well spread beyond California's borders. At the same time, he was in charge of maritime quarantine—not only at Angel Island, but also on the entire northern California coast. He had been supplied with extra personnel for these duties, but the aggregate responsibility was heavy. He had learned of a contract taken out on his life. He carried a loaded revolver, had a police guard, checked into hotels under an assumed name, and kept his launch ready for a quick escape to the quarantine station if needed.[36] Not to be forgotten was his family, isolated on Angel Island with four children, and lacking telephone connections.

Managing a plague epidemic, in fact, did not really fit into the job description of a quarantine officer. Kinyoun had fallen into it by chance, as an available and qualified person. And Wyman, worried as well, kept him on the job. The uproar of denials emanating from the governor, the press, and the business community had rendered the local health authorities and the city council essentially powerless.

Kinyoun's trial for contempt came up in June. The outcome in Kinyoun's mind was uncertain, and his telegrams to Wyman indicate that he felt quite alone, expressing doubts that everything was being done for his case. He confirmed this in the letter to Senator Cockrell.[37] The US attorney acting in his defense was also pessimistic. But in a surprise move the judge, possibly influenced by a chance encounter with Kinyoun during which the latter made clear the danger of plague and that he was acting under Wyman's orders, ruled that there had been no contempt of court.[38] Kinyoun's relief was profound, but he had little time for relaxation. Politicians and the press continued to hammer him. Bills were introduced in Sacramento to make it a crime to report a case of plague without confirmation by the California State Board of Health (controlled by Gage) and to prohibit the handling of cultures of the plague bacillus. The bills did not pass but indicated the mood.[39]

In December, Kinyoun vented his frustration in a long letter to Wyman. He complained that sanitation in Chinatown had not improved since plague first appeared, that the San Francisco Board of Health was without funds to accomplish meaningful inspections or cleaning, that doctors, often not competent, were making out death certificates without any autopsy, and that the press and political agencies were covering up the problem. He raged against the collector of customs for issuing of bills of health for ships departing to other US ports without due inspection. This risked spread to those ports. He added, pessimistically, "Whether the citizens of this city, as well as of the state, can be brought to a realization of the gravity of the situation, and be compelled to do something and eradicate this pest hole from San Francisco before it menaces still further the whole country is a debatable question. Probably no steps of a drastic nature, far-reaching in their consequences, or perfect in result, will be taken until a sufficient number of cases have occurred to cause consternation."[40] Shortly after the letter was sent, Governor Gage accused Kinyoun of injecting dead bodies with imported plague germs.[41]

In spite of press denials, plague continued to claim victims throughout the fall, some now outside Chinatown. The twenty-second case died on December 7. Wyman realized that he needed another approach to the standoff, and in early January 1901 he assigned Dr. Joseph H. White to investigate. White understood the problem promptly and suggested a tactful way out: an independent panel of experts to study the matter. This would provide a scientific opinion difficult to refute and push the issue to a higher and more public level. He also sympathized with Kinyoun's situation, writing, "Kinyoun exercises more self-restraint than I thought possible."[42]

For the expert opinion, Wyman chose three distinguished professors. Lewellys Barker, professor of anatomy at the University of Chicago; James Flexner, professor of pathology at the University of Pennsylvania Medical School; and Frederick Novy, professor of bacteriology at the University of Michigan, formed the team. Barker and Flexner had studied plague in Hong Kong (Barker had also seen it in India) and Novy had been in Budapest when Alexandre Yersin presented findings on plague bacilli from his Hong Kong experience.[43]

The committee of three arrived in San Francisco in January 1901. They set up a makeshift lab at city hall and went to work. Governor Gage had pressured the University of California to refuse bacteriology facilities to Dr. Novy, so Novy made arrangements in the back room of an under-taker's shop.[44] Concerned business owners agreed to help navigate other obstructions.[45] Additional cases had been accumulating, and while the commission was active six more residents died of plague, bringing the total to thirty-one deaths. Bacteriologic study of these cases confirmed the diagnosis of plague, and the San Francisco Plague Commission's (Plague Commission) report asserted clearly that an epidemic of plague existed in the city.[46] Twelve rats were caught and examined but none was found with plague, a surprise to the group. At least one of the group, Simon Flexner, concluded that rats played little if any role in plague trans-mission in San Francisco and that rats might even have some immunity to plague (later proved to be false).[47] The dismal condition of the Chinese living quarters was again noted.[48] In a separate article Barker added, as a gentle barb, that "a certain number of medical men, among them sev-eral of prominence" could not be convinced of the presence of plague.[49]

Governor Gage, as he heard reports of the findings, appealed to President McKinley for another investigation but was turned down. Gage finally agreed to the recommended sanitary measures (if cleared by him first), but he insisted that Kinyoun be relieved of duty and he wanted the findings of the Plague Commission kept quiet. Wyman, under pressure from a high-level group dispatched by Gage to Washington, agreed to the pact. He ordered his officers to proceed with case finding, isolation, and disinfection quietly and to avoid issuing alarming public statements.[50] White and Kinyoun were unhappy with the secrecy, but Wyman justified it by pointing out that no progress had been made with a confrontational stance.[51]

As the cleanup got under way, Kinyoun received a briefly worded order from Wyman, on April 6, reassigning him to a quarantine station in Detroit.[52] No explanation accompanied the order. Kinyoun was understandably distressed, believing that he had been unfairly treated by the local press, business interests, and politicians, and that he had not received sufficient recognition from Wyman. His dismissal was probably part of the bargain struck with Governor Gage, though the evidence is indirect.[53] Reading the dispatches to Wyman, it is evident that White, left to handle the outbreak, was also losing patience with the absurd situation.[54]

As White proceeded with the inspection and cleanup in Chinatown, he encountered obstacles quite familiar to Kinyoun. He faced continued denial by the governor and local politicians that plague existed. The California State Board of Health, under the thumb of Gage, was of no help and, in fact, was a hindrance.[55] The San Francisco Board of Health was the only group acknowledging plague but lacked authority and funds to accomplish much. Mayor Schmitz had tried to replace several members of the board but was thwarted by the courts. The city council continued to deprive the board of adequate funds and the newspapers hammered away with hostile commentary.

In April 1901 Wyman dispatched Passed Assistant Surgeon Rupert Blue to San Francisco to assist White. Blue, as assistant surgeon, had served for a short time as a boarding officer under Rosenau. Possessing valuable skills of tact and patience, he also benefitted from new developments. The results of the Plague Commission report were leaking out. Texas and Colorado had raised quarantines against California, harming business interests. Rumors of the loss of valuable military transport contracts circulated, worrying others engaged in business. Gage finally came to his senses, became somewhat more cooperative, and helped funnel needed funds for plague control. White and Blue set up an office and laboratory in San Francisco, finally relieving the MHS quarantine service from plague control duties and allowing it to concentrate on quarantine alone.

D. A. Carmichael returned as Kinyoun's short-term replacement, having recently dealt with a plague outbreak in Honolulu. He was replaced in May 1901 by Hugh Cummings. Now that others had assumed plague control measures in San Francisco, Cummings could avoid city politics and focus on quarantine. White, tired out from continuous hassle, was reassigned to Washington at his own request.[56]

Contrary to the Plague Commission report, others recognized the importance of rats in plague transmission, even though the exact role that they played was not clear. The San Francisco Department of Health, early in the outbreak, had placed poisoned fish down the sewers in Chinatown to kill rats.[57] Blue made further efforts to exterminate the rodents. But even Blue wearied and, having smoothed things over politically, returned at the end of the year to the Milwaukee Station from which he had come. MHS surgeon Mark White, who had been working with Rupert Blue (not to be confused with Joseph White, who had preceded Blue), subsequently instituted a formal program of rat extermination. Fortunately, no cases in other parts of California turned up.[58]

The epidemic accelerated the next year, with twenty-eight more residents succumbing during August, September, and October 1902. Several foreign ports set up quarantines against vessels from California. Health departments in other states, having lost patience with the fiasco, met in January 1903 and expressed outrage at the California authorities. They passed resolutions affirming that plague definitely existed in California and specifically charging Governor Gage and his state health department with obstructing antiplague measures.[59]

Other events helped mitigate the hostility to antiplague measures. A new governor, George Pardee, replaced Gage in early 1903. A physician himself but aware of public opinion, Pardee helped the health authorities behind the scenes. Rat-catching activities accelerated, and the city council decided to cooperate with added funds. Rupert Blue returned in May 1903. He further augmented rat-catching activities, promoted the use of rat poison, had more dwellings condemned and replaced with modern construction, and ordered leaky sewerage pipes repaired.[60] Of great importance, he implemented the cementing of basement floors, primarily in Chinatown, to prevent rats from nesting.[61]

Yet, during the remainder of 1903, plague refused to submit. New cases persistently came to light, seventeen of them between March and December. Anti-rat activities increased even more. In the twelve months ending on June 30, 1904, the plague teams cemented 139 basements, almost all of them in Chinatown, and continued to hunt down rats.[62] Finally, the measures proved their worth. Nine more cases trickled in during the first two months of 1904, but they were the last. The epidemic was finally over. A year later, a celebratory banquet was held in Rupert Blue's honor, after which he departed again, in April 1905.[63]

The final tally for the plague outbreak was 119 cases with 113 deaths, most of them among the Chinese.

Back on Angel Island, while the rat-catching and political squabbling continued in San Francisco, Hugh Cumming resumed reasonably normal quarantine duties. He faced new challenges, however. America was at war in the Philippines, an area where the health infrastructure was fragile and epidemic diseases commonplace. The United States had annexed Hawaii, a frequent stopping-off point for ships from Manila. The growing ship travel from these areas to California provided new opportunities for epidemic disease to reach San Francisco.

CHAPTER SEVEN

The Station in Middle Age

By 1901 PLAGUE HAD ERUPTED in Australia, China, Hawaii, Japan, New Zealand, the Philippines, and Thailand in the Pacific area; in India; and on the continents of Africa and South America. Even some European cities such as Liverpool, London, and Oporto had been invaded. Two years later it moved closer to California, becoming epidemic along the coast of Mexico.[1] India suffered horrific mortality, with deaths reaching well into the millions.[2] Trans-Pacific sea traffic from plague-infected areas was heavy and increasing. Fortunately, the idea that rats were important in the spread of plague was gaining acceptance, an idea that opened up a new approach to control. Guided by findings of an international conference in 1903, health authorities and shipping companies worked to rid ships of rats and keep them from crawling along ropes to access ships at the piers.[3] Blowing sulfur dioxide into holds, originally intended as a form of disinfection, now served to kill rats and insects as well as germs. The scientific community did not fully accept the role of the rat flea as a transmitter of plague until 1906, but fleas were under suspicion and were on the list of vermin to be kept off ships.[4] All vessels in San Francisco now used rat guards on their hawsers, kept hulls at least six feet from the dock, and raised gangplanks at night to prevent rats from disembarking or sneaking on board.[5] Ports elsewhere followed a similar program. In addition, ships grew larger and faster every year, now crossed the Pacific in fewer than eleven days and arrived even sooner from ports in Central and South America. The risk that a person could disembark in San Francisco with a disease still in the incubation phase grew steadily.[6]

In 1898 the United States went to war against Spain. Events during and after the war had a direct effect on the quarantine station. In nearby Cuba, the old nemesis of port cities along the southern coast, distressing numbers of American troops suffered and died from yellow fever. An Army research team, led by Walter Reed and using human volunteers, made history by establishing that a particular genus of mosquito, *Aedes*, transmitted the virus from person to person. Close personal contact was not the way that one victim infected others nor was there any poisonous miasma. The extermination of mosquitoes and interruption of their breeding cycle were now the methods used to prevent yellow fever. It is likely that earlier ship fumigation methods directed against yellow fever had been successful by ridding a vessel of mosquitoes and not by neutralizing miasmas or air carrying invisible germs.

In Havana, a city occupied by US forces during the war, General William Gorgas successfully eradicated *Aedes* mosquitoes by a combination of insecticide spraying and elimination of breeding sites. No longer would ships carry the virus from Havana to US shores. Ships from other Latin ports still posed risks, however, and quarantine measures depended on local conditions.

The war had additional repercussions on the other side of the globe. The Philippine Islands, acquired from Spain, were now an American possession. The United States annexed Hawaii as a territory shortly thereafter, making Honolulu a stopover port for many ships from the Philippines and the Asian coast. The Philippines was free of plague at the time of the American takeover in 1898, but not for long. A savage guerrilla war, pitting the American military against Philippine nationals who resisted occupation, had destabilized health control measures. Plague bacilli found their way into the abundant rat population in Manila and reached a prevalence among the rodents of 2 percent, considered close to epidemic levels.[7] Large numbers of people contracted the disease as well. In December 1899 plague reached across the Pacific to Honolulu. As it spread in Hawaii's largest city, authorities tried to confine it by instituting the selective burning of buildings, mainly in the Chinese area. Unexpectedly fierce winds, however, blew the fire out of control, destroying numerous homes and leaving thousands of Chinese homeless.[8] The tragedy was well known to the Chinese community in San Francisco and probably helped stiffen resistance to control measures.

In 1902 cholera, a disease that thrived where food and water are contaminated, reached the Philippines and exploded into a particularly severe epidemic that claimed more than 100,000 lives.[9] Tens of thousands of American soldiers were already in the Philippines and nearly 15,000 troops were stationed in San Francisco, training for overseas fighting.[10] A busy military and commercial traffic sprang up between Manila and San Francisco, supplementing the usual Asian traffic and creating favorable routes for disease transport. The Angel Island team watched these developments with some anxiety. Walter Wyman, following events from Washington, was also worried and took action.

The first goal was to bring the disease outbreaks in the new US possessions under control. Once that had been accomplished, it would be important to protect those territories from further importation of contagious disease. Congress renamed the MHS as the PHMHS in 1902.[11] The PHMHS opened quarantine stations in Honolulu and Manila, equipping them with all the apparatus found at the San Francisco station. Additional quarantine facilities were initiated on smaller Philippine and Hawaiian Islands.[12] The new stations supplied an extra layer of protection for San Francisco.

Cholera posed a special problem for the military. That disease had exploded on an astonishing twenty-three ships bound for California, most of them troop ships out of Manila, sending the GIs on board running to the overtaxed toilets. The infection usually found its way to the ship because a soldier had squirreled native food items on board just before departure.[13] To prevent further cholera outbreaks in midocean, vessels leaving Manila (primarily troopships) now waited in the harbor for five days before initiating a crossing, a period sufficient for a case in incubation to become evident. In addition, the military and the quarantine service struck an agreement that medical staff on returning troop ships could make decisions regarding quarantine without always consulting the MHS.

Several of the soldiers deployed overseas developed smallpox as they sailed home. The military had limited facilities available at the Presidio for smallpox and other contagious diseases. So as not to overburden the quarantine station, the Army built a separate detention camp on Angel Island, southeast of the quarantine station, to care for soldiers with quarantinable diseases, such as smallpox or cholera, and house those requiring isolation. As an added benefit, the MHS quarantine station was able to establish both telephone and telegraph connections through the Army camp and, for the first time, establish direct communication with the outside world.[14] The detention camp functioned until the end of hostilities, though it was not used very often and did not materially affect the MHS station.

At the same time, the California State Board of Health, concerned about the rising disease prevalence in the new territories and Asia, asked Wyman to advise the quarantine station to exercise still further vigilance against imported disease.[15] By 1901 Wyman had stationed medical personnel in several Asian ports, including Hong Kong, Yokohama, and Kobe. An important task of the officers stationed at foreign ports was to inspect and vaccinate passengers and often bathe them, fumigate ships and their cargo, and issue a clean bill of health before departure for America. Baggage that had been sterilized was labeled accordingly.[16]

The quarantine officer in San Francisco, boarding a ship with a valid bill of health, could grant pratique after a brief inspection and omit the usual disinfection of passengers and vessel. The availability of bills of health substantially reduced the workload. In fiscal year 1901, 62 vessels out of 1,087 were disinfected, and 3,572 passengers out of 71,048 inspected were disinfected.[17] By fiscal year 1904–5, as the PHMHS issued more bills of health overseas, the team disinfected only 25 out of 883 vessels (nearly half still using sail) and inspected only 2,460 passengers and crew out of 101,921. Smallpox was the only disease encountered that required quarantine during that time, though individual vessels had carried plague and yellow fever on board before arrival in San Francisco.[18] Disinfection of steerage passengers and crew entailed, as before, remaining in quarantine overnight for medical inspection and passing through the showers while clothing and luggage proceeded to the huge tanks for sterilization. The following day a launch ferried them to the mainland for immigration processing. According to Hugh Cumming, "With the present car system [small rail cars carrying belongings and certain cargo items to and from the giant sterilizers] put in by the station force it is believed that 2,000 persons can be handled in one day."[19] Selected cargoes, such as hides, animal hair, or rags, underwent disinfection as well. Cumming boasted that on one occasion 40,000 hides had been unbaled, disinfected in the giant sterilizers, and rebaled in three days.[20] For passengers held in quarantine, the shipping company paid $1.00 a day per person to the PHMHS.[21] The greater vigilance abroad kept the work in San Francisco at manageable levels. The efficient disinfection of steerage passengers and cargo from suspect ports and the provision of ships with bills of health at ports of origin were estimated to reduce the costs to shipowners by at least $2 million a year.[22]

When a ship arrived in San Francisco, a customs official boarded first, looking for contraband. Then came the quarantine officer looking for epidemic disease and, finally, somewhat later, another MHS officer boarded to medically examine immigrants, looking for physical problems that would affect suitability for immigration. The quarantine officer paid careful attention to swollen lymph glands and presence of fever, which were prominent clues to plague; the officer also checked for smallpox. All steerage passengers had their temperatures taken but cabin class passengers received more circumspect examination. Their temperatures were taken only if the ship had arrived in fewer than five or seven days (incubation periods established for cholera and plague, respectively) from an infected port, and thermometers for them were never used twice, even if washed in an antiseptic solution. The medical examination was also briefer. The inspector watched passengers walk, still clothed, taking temperatures if indicated. More detailed examination was undertaken only if disease was suspected, and the officer conducted it in private.[23]

By 1903 virtually all ships from Central and South American ports were suspect for plague as well as cholera and yellow fever, a triple threat. "The passed [sic] year has been one of daily anxiety and apprehension for the quarantine officer at this port," wrote Hugh Cumming in July 1903. "During the past year, two hundred and fifty-six vessels have arrived at this port from ports where cholera or plague or both prevail and fifty-two from yellow fever ports."[24] (In reality, yellow fever was a small risk since the proper mosquito vector probably did not exist in or near San Francisco, though this was not known.) The lazaret continued to harbor smallpox victims. Medical officers were in place at Guayaquil, Ecuador; and Callao, Peru, to report on health conditions and issue bills of health if possible. They eased the work at home.[25]

The composition of passenger traffic was also changing. The Chinese Exclusion Act of 1882 had severely reduced the flow of Chinese immigration. Chinese passengers since then were usually those born in the United States (and their progeny), persons with exemptions from the act's restrictions, or previous residents possessing proper documents.[26] They generally belonged to a more affluent category, usually traveled in cabin class, and, if placed in quarantine, lodged in the white house, which were the nicer quarters now available for them on Angel Island. And, as noted, medical examination was more nuanced and tactful.[27]

As fewer Chinese laborers arrived by sea, Japanese workers filled the gap. Japan had resisted emigration in the past, but a demand for farm labor in Hawaii led to reconsideration of the policy. A contract between the Japanese and Hawaiian governments in 1886 allowed Japanese citizens to emigrate to the islands for farm labor, and many did. After Hawaii was annexed to the United States in 1898, immigration of Japanese from Hawaii to the United States was possible, and higher American wages induced many to try their luck in California. Direct immigration from Japan also increased until 1907, when an unwritten agreement between the Japanese and US governments restricted it.[28] Japanese shipping companies, meanwhile, had moved in to capture a portion of the Pacific passenger and commercial traffic.[29] Wyman stationed PHMHS officers in key Japanese ports who tried to ensure that clean ships with healthy passengers arrived at the American coast.

In 1901 shock waves pulsed through the nation when a professed anarchist gunned down President McKinley. As the country mourned, officers at the quarantine station wore black armbands for thirty days.[30] McKinley's vice president and successor, Theodore Roosevelt, urged Congress to pass a new immigration law, specifically to exclude anarchists. The new legislation, the Act to Regulate the Immigration of Aliens into the United States, passed in March 1903, also reaffirmed a prior immigration act of 1891 that denied entry to the United States of immigrants with "a loathsome or dangerous contagious disease," with insanity or "idiocy" (mental retardation), or with various medical or social conditions liable to render them a public charge or nuisance. Included in the latter categories were prostitutes, criminals, beggars, paupers, polygamists, and those with disabling physical conditions. The new act also continued an 1891 provision that PHMHS officers medically examine the immigrants.[31] Wyman ordered the quarantine station to add immigrant inspections to the quarantine duties, work previously done in San Francisco by contract physicians.

The PHMHS physicians' assignment was to examine immigrants and report on their medical findings, leaving judgments to the US Bureau of Immigration on whether an applicant should be admitted or rejected. Medical decisions could be appealed to a medical board consisting of three physicians.[32] Nationality was not to play a role in decisions, and cabin class passengers received a more courteous examination.[33] Although the examiners were PHMHS officers under loose supervision of the commander of the quarantine station, they sent their reports directly to the Bureau of Immigration.[34] Since the immigration authorities had no office on the island (the immigration station was not opened on Angel Island until 1910), the officers performed the examinations on incoming ships, using ad hoc arrangements to examine up to a few hundred people at a time and complete the necessary paperwork. To cope with the increased workload of immigrant examinations, Wyman assigned an extra officer to the station. The officer was generally on duty from sunrise to sunset.[35]

Wyman composed an instruction guide for examiners. The manual discussed methods of examination and clarified certain diseases and terms. Diseases placed in Class A were automatic grounds for exclusion. Class A diseases consisted of (a) dangerous contagious diseases, defined as trachoma (an infectious eye disease—see below) and active tuberculosis of the lungs with the organism demonstrable in a sputum specimen; and (b) loathsome diseases, of which there were four categories: (a) favus (a contagious scalp disease caused by a fungus); (b) gonorrhea, syphilis, and leprosy; (c) insanity; and (d) idiocy (a condition now called cognitive disability or dementia). Class B conditions comprised a hodgepodge of diseases and deformities that were likely to result in the immigrant becoming a public charge. These included such things as valvular heart disease, disabling arthritis, cancer, senility, blindness, and so forth, and did not necessarily result in automatic exclusion.[36] The quarantinable diseases—smallpox, cholera, plague, yellow fever, and typhus—were, of course, separately diagnosed by the quarantine officer and did not apply to immigration criteria.

Trachoma, branded as a loathsome disease, had become a common sight at the quarantine station. It is an infectious disease of the eyes, passed from person to person by direct contact and by flies, and flourishes in areas of poverty and crowding. The world of antiquity knew it well, having recorded its existence in ancient Egypt as well as ancient Greece and Rome.[37] Napoleon's soldiers stationed in Egypt suffered almost universally from it. Trachoma is believed to have entered the United States through immigration.[38] The causative organism is a species of *Chlamydia*, a variant of one that infects the genital tract. Initially the eyes are reddened and inflamed. If untreated, the continued inflammation leads to gradual scarring of the lids and cornea. Scarring may deform the lids so that the eyelashes turn in toward the surface of the eye and damage the cornea. Eventually blindness ensues as corneal scarring renders the cornea opaque. California officials feared that afflicted immigrants would disseminate it, especially in schools. Ellis Island in New York had a wide experience with the malady.[39]

Since science had not uncovered the causative organism by 1901, the diagnosis of trachoma depended on a clinical examination of the eyes, a process that included everting the upper lid. Thickening of the eye-lids and dullness of the cornea, characteristic of later stages, rendered the diagnosis fairly certain. Medical examiners often disagreed, however, over milder cases that presented few telltale signs. Such cases frequently resulted in an appeal to a medical board.[40] The conflicting opinions frustrated the boards, and at one point Wyman ordered the Angel Island examining officer to travel to Vancouver to confer with a fellow officer and agree on diagnostic criteria. (PHMHS officers were posted in Canada to inspect immigrants passing through a Canadian port on their way to California).[41]

Japanese passengers had the highest incidence of trachoma and the incidence detected by medical officers was rising. On one ship arriving from Hawaii in 1905, 155 cases turned up out of 909 steerage passengers.[42] The PHMHS officer, Hugh Cumming, requested the companies owning the vessels to urge ship doctors to exert more care in screening passengers before departure in order to reduce deportations. He also favored putting trachoma in the same category as leprosy, meaning immediate deportation.[43] That request was declined, however.[44] The California State Health Department also considered refusing entry to all trachoma victims.[45] The disease was believed to have arisen in the United States through immigration and there was a widespread fear that it would make its way into the school classrooms and workplaces.[46] Stories in the press about the increase in trachoma engendered wider calls for limits on Japanese immigration, intensifying an already pervasive atmosphere of discrimination.[47]

Mild or indeterminate cases, because of difficulty in diagnosis, were often held for observation. Due to the lack of a suitable facilities to house suspicious cases, however, indeterminate cases were often passed through. In the 1903–4 reporting year, 208 passengers were certified as having trachoma, but only 8 passengers were deported.[48] By 1909 most cases diagnosed with trachoma were brought before a medical board of inquiry to confirm the diagnosis. At the same time, arrivals with trachoma dropped considerably. The report for 1911 indicates that eleven immigrants were deported for trachoma.[49] A factor restricting deportations was a court ruling that "aliens having become domiciled in the United States and returning from visits abroad" could not be deported.[50] Such returning legal residents made up a fair number of cases. In addition, the increased examinations of immigrants in their ports of origin before departure culled out many cases that would have arrived at San Francisco and else-where.[51] One of the PHMHS officers contracted trachoma during his duties as inspector of immigrants.[52] That was rare, however.[53]

Some immigrants sought a method to outwit the trachoma inspections—adrenalin.[54] Passengers dropped adrenalin solution in their eyes that would constrict the small blood vessels on the surface, making the eye appear less inflamed than it really was. The press carried a story of an unscrupulous ship surgeon (on the SS *Doric*) suspected of selling adrenalin solution to passengers.[55]

The other category of dangerous contagious disease, tuberculosis, was certifiable as such if typical symptoms were present and the organism could be found in the sputum. X-rays were a novelty at the time, intro-duced in 1895, and played no role in screening. In the loathsome disease category, syphilis was grounds for deportation, while the immigrant with gonorrhea could be allowed in if treatment was successful.[56]

Medical examinations often yielded indefinite results. Temporary ill-nesses or illnesses of uncertain diagnosis were examples, and they caused delays. Passengers found with pneumonia or other serious problems went to the San Francisco PHMHS hospital, located on the Presidio, for treat-ment. Those with lighter ailments, including mild or early trachoma, were usually held for treatment in hopes of clarifying the diagnosis or achiev-ing recovery, rather than resorting to automatic deportation. A wooden structure, known as the detention shed, located on the PMSS pier, served as the holding area for the borderline cases. It was a building with an unappetizing history that began with the Spanish-American War.

At the outbreak of the Spanish-American War, the military comman-deered almost all passenger ships for troop transportation, leaving no floating vessels on which to hold immigrants temporarily. The PMSS, the main San Francisco carrier, converted the upper story of a two-story office building located on their large pier, Pier 40, into a detention shed, a title retained long after the war was over.[57] The press labeled it the Hotel Mongolia.[58] Newspaper reports indicate that the space was dirty, overcrowded, and that attempted escapes were not uncommon.[59] The commissioner general of immigration at the time complained that "the detention shed there should be abolished forthwith. Chinese are human beings and are entitled to humane treatment, and this is something they do not receive under present conditions."[60] Some detainees harbored dis-eases such as tuberculosis and trachoma while they sat in close quarters that were ideal conditions for further spread. The immigration station opened on Angel Island in 1910 and replaced the detention shed.

Miscellaneous other, less-frequent, quarantine problems challenged the PHMHS. Unusual ship cargoes raised uncertainties about the methods of, or the need for, disinfection. For instance, what to do with nine thousand pounds of human hair, or on another occasion a shipment of forty cases of human hair.[61] They were treated with naphthalene before being allowed in.[62] Shipments of small dark cubes in boxes labeled "medicine" aroused curiosity. The cubes turned out to be dried human feces, used in some way (never determined) for medicinal purposes. On bacteriological examination, they were almost sterile and were passed through. The PHMHS laboratory studied a variety of dried foods and concluded that they were generally safe.[63] Medicines, in general, were forwarded to the Pure Food and Drug Bureau Laboratory (created after the Pure Food and Drug Act of 1906) for examination.[64] Shipments of bone meal or rags from India and the Middle East were infrequent and required at least sixty days at sea or some form of disinfection.[65] Other unusual items included eggs buried in mud, water lily bulbs, and various types of dried fish. In general, the inspectors were accommodating, refusing only articles reasonably believed to be unsafe.

In October 1909 a human corpse arrived from Victoria, British Colombia, unaccompanied by any papers. The ship's manifest listed the body as "merchandise," though a second manifest labeled it as "natural history specimen." The quarantine officer ordered the body to remain on board, pending an inspection or submission of a death certificate, but when he arrived the next day, he found the coffin empty.[66] The body was never found.

Surveying the broader picture, in 1903 Cumming summarized the life and work at the Angel Island Quarantine Station. The facility was humming along efficiently in many respects, but there were grievances. Crumbling linoleum, absent window coverings in staff bedrooms, inadequate furniture, broken iceboxes, and the like were complaints that Cumming forwarded to Wyman. The only horse on the station was old, worn out, and needed to be replaced. Motorized vehicles were still a dream. A horse and cart still hauled furniture, coal, garbage, and supplies uphill or downhill.[67]

Two years later, though, improvements brightened the station. Additional new buildings, pushed laterally by limited flat space, crept

up the hills surrounding the Hospital Cove area. They afforded pleasant
views, but it still required effort to transport supplies uphill. By 1905 thirty
buildings covered about twenty-five acres on the station. Many gleamed
with new paint, new toilets, and electric lighting. Eighteen personnel, in
addition to the medical officers and the boarding crew, staffed the station.[68] By 1907 thirty-five buildings were scattered over thirty-five acres. A
new contagious disease hospital to care for cases of diphtheria, smallpox,
and measles originating in other government facilities (such as a nearby
naval training station) met an additional need.

Living quarters grew more comfortable. The medical officer in charge
and his family could relax in a larger house with a living room, dining
room, kitchen, library, and four bedrooms. The assistant surgeon and the
pharmacist enjoyed a similar house with two bedrooms. Others lodged
in smaller quarters.[69] Outdoor verandas on residential buildings allowed
the staff to enjoy the balmy summer and fall climate in the shelter of the
surrounding hills. New housing offered comfortable facilities, previously
not available, for the cabin class passengers. The cabin class passengers,
increasing in numbers, objected to life with the hoi polloi in the barracks,
and Washington heeded their complaints. When the SS *Umatilla* arrived
in 1908, carrying a case of smallpox, the available comfortable space was
inadequate for 189 second-class cabin passengers (a category above steerage class). They ended up in the barracks where, according to Cumming,
"I have now in the Chinese and Japanese barracks aged women and little
children who sleep on bunks without adequate cover, use troughs for
toilets, and eat on the floor."[70] Cumming's complaint brought money
for better facilities and highlighted conditions in the more primitive barracks for steerage class. In addition, the barracks, lit with kerosene lamps,
were a potential firetrap. Cracks between the wall planks rendered them
drafty and precluded efficient fumigation.[71] A load of American soldiers
returning from the Philippines who required quarantine occasionally
overcrowded the facility.

Weather could prove damaging. During a storm in November 1901,
a heavy surf hurled a station launch onto a rock near shore. Two crewmembers were on board, one of whom died of injuries that evening.[72]
Another storm in January blew so severely that the *Omaha* broke its
anchor chain, drifting to San Pablo Bay.[73] Three years later, an eighty-
mile-an-hour gale blew the *Omaha* once more off its mooring. It took a
team of three tugs, with engines at full power and operating at high tide,

to finally free it from a tenacious muddy bottom.[74] Other storms damaged the sea wall, blew roofs off two buildings and the blacksmith's shop, flattened or uprooted several trees, and undermined roads and paths.[75]

Periodic freshwater shortages continued, in spite of a deeper well. Saltwater for cleaning the bathhouses and barracks helped, temporarily.[76] Electric lighting appeared in more and more buildings, but coal remained the primary fuel to power lighting, cooking, sterilizing, and heat. On the mainland, by contrast, the transition to less-expensive oil was well under way. Iceboxes, supplied with regular ice deliveries, were now available to preserve meat and other perishables. Water closets were generally in use except in the Chinese Barracks. The telephone underwater cable was severed in early 1904, and a new one could not be laid until early 1906, a great inconvenience that resulted in delays and frustration. Ship captains wanting to send a message to the station had to send it to the mainland first, from where it went by launch or mail to the station. They waited up to two days for a reply.[77]

A new horse finally replaced the old one but proved to be temperamental. On one occasion the horse bucked suddenly, throwing a cart and its driver into the Bay. After two more similar episodes the PHMHS officer pleaded for a tamer animal—a mule.[78] New horses were supplied instead.

The boarding launch, the *George Sternberg*, originally built as a disinfecting tug, was showing its age. Its worn appearance and slow speed made it the butt of jokes on the Bay, something the staff complained about.[79] Money for a replacement finally came through in 1905. The new boarding vessel, the *Neptune* (renamed *Argonaut* a short time later), was a second-hand vessel whose appearance did not inspire confidence. The interior was dirty. The plumbing was "the most remarkable ever seen"— most of the toilet flush emptied into the bilge. Washbasins were broken or dirty, the stove badly worn, and the oven damaged. Deck hoses were decayed and unusable, the mattresses filthy and filled with corn shucks, and in the after cabin lay a carpet saturated with saltwater, tobacco juice, and engine room grease.[80] The *Neptune* (*Argonaut*) was, however, larger and more powerful, able to contend with the rough seas common on the Bay and the budget allowed for the needed improvements. It burned coal, though eventually was converted to oil in 1909.

Labor difficulties hampered efficient use of the boarding vessel. The firemen who shoveled the coal worked for meager wages. They put in fourteen-hour days with no leave, in contrast to a ten-hour day with regular monthly leave on tugboats.[81] According to Surgeon Hobdy (who followed Cumming), the firemen were "third class men, rough, profane, and many times bums whose sole ideas seem to be to hang on till they reach payday, then we lose their services either from drunkenness or from insubordination while they are in a semi-intoxicated condition."[82] On another occasion, Hobdy could not persuade a cook to stay on the job. "More than once it looked as if everybody except the Pilot and Engineer would leave and the boat would have to go out of commission."[83] The underlying problem, he grumbled, was the low pay.

Working on the boarding steamer could also be hazardous. Sometimes a rope ladder was the only means available to board a ship. In rough seas a rope ladder swayed perilously, and in rain it was wet and slippery. The officer climbing the ladder was usually weighed down with several volumes of paperwork and hundreds of thermometers. The heaving gunwale of the boarding launch could catch a rung of the ladder and snap the rope. On one occasion a deckhand's hand was crushed between the gunwale of the boarding launch and the ship's hull, and on another, an officer fell backward onto the boarding launch from an improperly secured ladder. Equipment occasionally tumbled into the deep.[84] One deckhand was lost overboard, but the reason why he fell never came to light.[85]

The substandard pay of personnel, the disinclination to invest in oil, the delays in making repairs, and similar delays all stemmed from budgetary limits set by Congress. Receipts, even for small amounts, were often queried. In December 1905 Wyman made a request to reduce the number of personnel, a reduction the station could ill afford.[86]

Pollution of the waters of the Bay was increasing dramatically. Unrestricted sewage runoff and industrial effluents darkened the water, and oil slick covered the surface extensively. Even sewage from the quarantine station went into the Bay. The filth was so severe that it was difficult to keep the *Argonaut*'s hull clean. Quoting Hobdy, "The water of the bay at our berth is so filthy from sewers and crude oil, that its use [for cleaning] is out of the question most of the time."[87] The crew drew freshwater from the station's well to clean the hull, limiting the supply for other purposes. Measures to limit pollution in the Bay were decades in the future.

The launch *Bacillus*, used for errands to and from the station, also grew old and leaky, becoming a "menace to her crew and a disgrace to the Service [MHS]."[88] Hobdy even asked permission to purchase food from the military post exchange at Ft. McDowell next door rather than risk a ride in the launch to the mainland.[89] Orders finally came through for a replacement launch.

The vigilance of the quarantine officers prevented further introduction of epidemic disease into San Francisco in the years after the plague epidemic; in spite of limited budgets and social isolation it functioned efficiently. The medical officers were, on the other hand, powerless to resist a different threat, that of plague arising from within. The plague bacillus, apparently vanished from San Francisco, had, in reality, continued life surreptitiously. Rats and their germ-ridden fleas continued to inhabit cozy nests inside basements, stables, and warehouses in San Francisco. Inevitably, the germs they carried made their way back to humans. This time, though, the task confronting the quarantine officers was quite different: how to prevent plague from leaving San Francisco and moving by sea vessel to another port.

CHAPTER EIGHT

Plague Returns

EARLY IN THE MORNING of April 18, 1906, a rumbling noise startled the residents of San Francisco. Movements of the ground underneath the city rocked houses and buildings and threw sleepy residents off balance as they climbed out of bed. Rushing outside, the startled populace encountered chasms lacerating the streets, saw buildings collapsing among a hail of bricks and stones, and witnessed subterranean water and sewerage pipes being wrenched apart. Devastating fires broke out, sweeping through the tottering buildings. The fire department, racing to quench the flames, found itself helpless in the face of destroyed water mains. Chinatown, with its rickety structures, suffered severe damage. The fires, pushed along by vigorous winds, raged relentlessly, incinerating the houses and buildings unlucky enough to stand in the way. The greater part of San Francisco ended in ruins. Frightened inhabitants ran for safety, thousands of them crowding onto ferries heading for Oakland or Marin County. At least 30,000 people were suddenly homeless.

Tent cities sprang up haphazardly. The city faced critical shortages of food, water, sanitation, shelter, and, to some extent, law and order. Ferries continued to evacuate frightened residents, extra police were deputized, and the Army, under General Funston, took early control. Mayor Schmitz, his reputation tarnished by the corrupt administration around him, rose unexpectedly to the occasion and also assumed a leadership role. The firefighters eventually brought the inferno under control, the damage was assessed, and before long rebuilding began. Fortunately, harm to the San Francisco waterfront was not as severe as in the city at large. The Navy was called into action and hosed the waterfront copiously with saltwater, limiting the damage.[1] In a short time, ships were able to dock as before, a vital step needed to accommodate the supplies of lumber, building materials, and food flowing into the harbor.

The earthquake shook Angel Island, causing moderate damage to the quarantine station. Roofs, chimneys, walls, furniture, and certain provisions were damaged to varying degrees, but no fires compounded the earthquake's effects. The launch and its rails were damaged. The boarding vessel, the *Argonaut,* still functioned and aided the ferries in transporting terrified and homeless refugees to nearby shores. It also delivered much-needed supplies to the ad hoc refugee camps in San Francisco and, with an armed guard on board, pressed tugboats into doing the same. Repair work at the station began shortly after the earthquake. In contrast to the havoc and misery of the city, the quarantine service continued to function after only a brief pause.[2]

Eight months later, the following December, the station suffered again, this time from a horrific storm, said to be the worst in twenty years. The fierce winds felled trees, ripped most of the shingles off the so-called Chinese Barracks, carried away a chimney flue, and shattered several windows. Rain poured through mutilated roofs and, on the *Omaha,* damaged the underlying machinery. A loosed mooring punched a hole in the launch.[3] In San Francisco, the havoc of the storm compounded that of the earthquake. Roofs were carried off, partly reconstructed buildings toppled again, flying debris battered pedestrians and cars, basements and sewerage lines flooded, and some streets, such as Fillmore, resembled rivers. In the tent encampments, the frail canvases providing primitive shelter blew away, leaving numerous hapless inhabitants in the open air.[4]

The station recovered from these problems relatively easily, but rebuilding the city took time. Thousands were homeless, the tent cities continued to fester, and sanitation facilities improved at a slow pace. Wyman was concerned about the health consequences and dispatched Rupert Blue, instrumental in the plague outbreak a few years earlier, to investigate. A newly arrived officer at the quarantine station developed typhoid fever, having possibly been exposed in San Francisco.[5] In late April, a single, but nonfatal, case of plague turned up in Oakland, across the Bay from San Francisco. It probably came from the ground squirrel population that was now infected. Preoccupied with earthquake damages, the media paid little attention. But Blue knew that the earthquake had left San Francisco vulnerable. He also knew that residents of Oakland had reported seeing dead ground squirrels, though, when he investigated, he was unable to find any.[6] He worried that plague might break out in the refugee camps in San Francisco, which were often in proximity to rat-infested areas and suffered from inadequate sanitation. Fortunately, no plague appeared.

However, the disease was closing in from abroad. Three cases of plague surfaced in Honolulu in August of 1906 and additional cases appeared in 1907, alarming the San Francisco station as well as the California State Board of Health.[7] Added to that was evidence that quarantine practices in Honolulu were deficient, prompting the California State Board of Health to consider dispatching a commission to investigate. W. C. Hobdy, station chief in 1906, drew up recommendations to allay these fears and the Hawaii station implemented them soon after.[8] As a result, ships from Honolulu now carried reliable documentation of antiplague measures, obviating the need to repeat the procedures in San Francisco.

Plague transported by sea did not penetrate Angel Island's quarantine barriers in the years after the epidemic of 1900, but the pestilence onshore, only temporarily subdued, had been spreading through the San Francisco rodent population. In May 1907 doctors in the San Francisco MHS Hospital cared for a seaman desperately ill with a raging fever and swollen lymph glands. After a brief but stormy illness that took his life, an autopsy revealed unmistakable signs of plague. Hurried inquiries uncovered that the seaman had served on a tugboat plying coastal ports and, furthermore, that the craft had just departed again, heading north and towing a barge. As the authorities chased it down, the ill-fated vessel struck a rock, sending the tug rapidly to the bottom. The crew, scrambling for their lives, managed to reach the still-floating barge. All survived and none showed any signs of plague. The matter seemed closed.[9]

About ten weeks later, an Italian couple in the North Beach area of San Francisco fell ill with fever and painful, inflamed glands, typical of plague. One of the couple died. Other cases followed, soon in accelerating numbers.[10] In the MHS Hospital another seaman died, thought to have pneumonia. At autopsy the lungs proved to be filled with plague bacilli. An immediate search located his ship, the *Samoa,* and, according to Surgeon Hobdy, "She swarms with vermin and while no one on board is ill, dead rats have been found." He ordered the boat and crew into quarantine, and had the surviving rats killed. No one developed fever.[11]

But the writing was on the wall. One month later, plague attacked twenty-five San Franciscans, thirteen fatally, and this time the sufferers came from areas in San Francisco that previously had been unaffected. Notably, only one case so far was Chinese, and that case was the president of the Chinese Six Companies, not a poor man. The concrete that had been copiously poured into Chinatown to create rat-proof basements had paid off. The enterprising rats had moved to other more hospitable spots, and to the waterfront.

Even in the San Francisco General Hospital, patients under treatment for unrelated problems came down with plague. The General Hospital, built in 1872 on Potrero Street in the Mission District to serve the poor of the city, had somehow survived the 1906 earthquake. In the wake of the earthquake, a city-wide typhoid epidemic created a further strain on the chronically overburdened facility, overtaxing its resources. When the first cases of plague emerged, an inspection revealed the hospital to be swarming with rats. All patients, except those with plague, were immediately evacuated to other facilities and the hospital remained open to serve only plague patients. A rat-proof fence went up around the grounds to prevent rodents from escaping into the community.[12]

Politicians were more cooperative this time. The mayor, Edward Taylor, who took office in July 1907, telegraphed President Theodore Roosevelt for help, who in turn notified Wyman. The San Francisco Department of Health leaned on Station Chief Hobdy for assistance, since he had the best laboratory. Hobdy, already fully immersed in quarantine duties, dispatched a telegram to Wyman. He asked for help controlling "bumpkin," the code word used for plague to avoid alarming anyone seeing telegraphed messages. Wyman acted without delay. He dispatched the experienced Rupert Blue once more to assume plague control measures. Blue's plague skills and easygoing personality, instrumental in the last epidemic, were well known by this time to San Franciscans.

On arrival, Blue, now armed with more complete knowledge of the role of rats and their fleas in plague transmission, set to work. There was no sign that the recent cases of plague had slipped into San Francisco through the quarantine net. Rather, infections in the rat population had simmered at a low level and were now exploding, aided by the chaos in the wake of the earthquake.

Blue's team set up a laboratory and office on Fillmore Street, transferred the plague diagnostic facilities back from Angel Island, and hired rat-catchers and inspectors. He divided the city into districts, each with a medical officer who carried out inspections to ascertain sanitary conditions, locate rat habitats, and find cases of plague. The federal government contributed $50,000 to the overstretched city funds. And this time the business community and the press, with the exception of the *San Francisco Chronicle*, were cooperative. The mayor appointed a Citizens'

Health Committee, composed primarily of business owners and physicians, that supervised and financed much of the work.[13] The city administration passed appropriate ordinances as needed.

The medical officers roaming through San Francisco encountered alarming conditions, partly resulting from the earthquake. Though the Red Cross had set up clean, sanitary camps for many of the homeless, others lived in clusters of dilapidated, makeshift shacks surrounded by open latrines, garbage, swarms of flies, and general filth, all of that creating ideal havens for rats. Damaged pipes deprived several city areas of sewerage connections. Outside the camps, rat-infested basements, litter-lined streets, and homes harboring either pigs or cows were common sights. Garbage collection was unreliable. Horse stables and chicken yards, ideal sites for rat nesting, were scattered through the city.

All establishments conducive to rat habitation were cleaned, fumigated, and rendered rat-proof by various means including lining floors with concrete. Efficient garbage collection and mending of sewerage lines were other important measures. Teams of workers set rat traps and laid poison. They received a daily wage plus a bounty of ten cents per dead rat and earned promotions or demotions depending on their performance. The laboratory examined all rats caught by trappers and recorded their location. If a rat was infected, the teams made special efforts to clean and rat-proof that location. Overall, estimates were that about a million rats were killed through the combined efforts of all parties.[14]

The waterfront, too, was crawling with rats. One or more could easily slip on board a vessel tied alongside and hitch a ride to the next landing. When Hobdy opened the door of an abandoned stable on one of the piers, he encountered swarms of rats, some of them dead with plague. Another shed was in the same condition.[15] To quote Hobdy, "Never in the history of San Francisco have there been so many rats on the waterfront. This is the consensus of opinion of all the 'waterfronters.' There is further a marked mortality among these rats."[16]

The challenge was to ensure that all vessels leaving the port of San Francisco were rat-free and plague-free. Without prompt intervention, the spread of plague from San Francisco to distant ports was almost certain. The challenge was formidable. Numerous small vessels crisscrossed the Bay on a daily basis, ferrying both goods and people. They moved from the city to landings all around the Bay, motoring up the Sacramento River and cruising along the Pacific coast. Every landing spot was a potential destination for infected rats. Furthermore, failure to police traffic out of the Golden Gate would inevitably invite quarantine measures against San Francisco by other states and countries. During the previous outbreak of 1900, denial of plague's existence and local political resistance had generated a few such quarantines. It was probably pure luck that plague did not escape to other ports at the time.

Blue left it to the quarantine service to police the boat traffic. The California State Board of Health asked Hobdy to draw up procedures, which he did. He then contacted Wyman with his plans, asking for approval.[17] Wyman gave his approval without hesitation and Hobdy issued a directive ordering that all coastal vessels lying "at any dock along the coast" be fumigated at once to kill rats and observe rat precautions.[18] The California State Board of Health issued its own order that all vessels "lying at dock anywhere on the coast" were to observe rat precautions and be fumigated on leaving the dock.[19] Wyman soon extended fumigations to include all vessels leaving San Francisco for Canada, Hawaii, and Mexico.[20] A little later he added the Philippines and Panama.

The magnitude of the task far exceeded the capabilities of the station's fumigation launch. Any vessel on the Bay with an enclosed space big enough to hold rats was a candidate for a dose of sulfur dioxide. This encompassed hundreds of craft—sailing vessels, ferries, and steamers. Fumigation on that scale required an approach of a greater magnitude, and teams of fumigators were hired to accomplish the task. They placed Dutch oven pans on each and every vessel needing fumigation. In the pans they deposited roughly two and a half pounds of sulfur for every thousand cubic feet of treated space. A small amount of wood alcohol was then poured over the sulfur and a match applied. The burning sulfur emitted copious sulfur dioxide fumes that filled the space in cargo holds, galleys, dining rooms, staterooms, and most other compartments. All hatches, portholes, and doors were closed and the malignant fumes kept in the sealed spaces for eight to twelve hours. An authorized inspector supervised the work and, upon completion, issued a certificate that the captain retained as a seal of approval for his next docking. The certificate expired in six weeks, after which a new fumigation and certificate were required.[21] The California State Department of Health weighed in and included all ferries and other small craft in its own regulations, hiring state inspectors to supervise the work.[22] The usual docking precautions (lying six feet off the pier, rat guards on the hawsers, etc.) were enforced for all vessels.

Fumigating so many vessels was a tall order. The project began on September 2, 1907. Hobdy purchased ten tons of sulfur, along with Dutch oven pans and other equipment. For the labor, he hired forty men and provided them with sleeping and eating facilities. The *George Sternberg*, ailing but still afloat, underwent hasty repairs and was entered into service. The *Argonaut* was pulled from boarding duty to carry fumigators to larger ships and to patrol the waterfront, while revenue cutter boats took over the more usual duties of quarantine boarding and inspection of incoming ships. The PHMHS officer assigned to the medical inspection of immigrants was transferred to help with fumigation, causing backups in the immigration process. Ship owners also complained of delays. The California State Department of Health fumigated vessels operating on inland waterways and placed personnel for inspection at inland ports, areas outside the jurisdiction of the PHMHS. To protect the remaining coast, Hobdy asked Wyman to urge the corresponding ports in Washington and Oregon to take similar rat elimination measures. He cited the recent example of Sydney, Australia, where plague had spread along routes plied by local boats.[23] Wyman complied.

A serious problem was what to do with smaller craft that visited minor docks where inspectors were often absent. They included ferries and small craft with irregular delivery schedules. Without agents to enforce rules, skippers were less likely to comply with them. Hobdy had only three officers, hardly enough to supervise the entire waterfront. Put bluntly by Hobdy, "The Bureau [the Quarantine Division of the PHMHS] by its telegram of August 26th has more than tripled my work and yet seems to expect me to do this increased work with the same force that I had for regular quarantine work before the telegram came. It is an impossibility."[24]

But Hobdy carried on. Wyman sent one extra medical officer and authorized Hobdy to hire local doctors as temporary fumigation supervisors.[25] The local doctors showed little interest, though, as Hobdy cynically noted, writing that they refused because of low pay.[26] A few eventually signed on, though, and the state health department contributed more personnel. By late September, Hobdy had enough laborers to apply fumigations to all craft leaving San Francisco, including those going up the Sacramento River. Local craft with frequent runs, such as ferries, were fumigated every two weeks, others once a month. A total of 242 vessels were disinfected and certified during the first month of operations, September 1907, a monumental achievement considering the meager personnel and enormous confusion. The number roughly doubled the next month. A few cases of plague had turned up in Oakland, another busy port across the Bay, and the same fumigation measures were applied.[27] New rat-proof storage bins for cargo were erected on piers to prevent rats from sneaking into otherwise porous containers of goods about to be shipped elsewhere.

Wyman wanted comprehensive reports, including figures on rats killed, expenses, numbers and types of craft certified, and the like, for future study.[28] At first, the rat counts were incomplete—the fumigating crews had no time to find and count rats and the captains were uninterested because of the delay entailed and through fear that the numbers might reflect badly on their ship. Eventually, the crews counted the dead rodents more carefully and the results made it clear that the rat populations on most vessels were dropping. Occasional exceptions were those that traveled to certain South American ports where regulations were lax.

Oil tankers posed a particular problem. They were no exception in harboring rats, but rats avoided the oil-filled holds and sought refuge in the cabins, galleys, and other compartments. Normally, tankers tied up to the hulk *Omaha* for fumigation, whose flexible hosing forced sulfur dioxide into the infested compartments. However, the hose was so worn out and leaky that using it was "little more than a pretense."[29] The alternative was to light fires in sulfur pots, the method used on other ships, to fumigate the compartments. But lighting fires on a vessel carrying 16,000 barrels of oil did not appeal to the quarantine officer and horrified the captains, the owners, and the marine insurance companies. Hobdy lit fires anyway, though he soon backed off at the insistence of ship agents, while he pleaded to Wyman for new hoses.

Amazingly, the Wyman's Quarantine Division demurred, objecting to the cost of the hoses. Desperate and exasperated, Hobdy turned to the state health department, asking them to intervene:

> The question resolves itself into this: The Bureau says, "Disinfect, but you can't have any hose." The owners, agents, underwriters, and inspectors say, "You must not use pans." And I want to know how it is to be done. I know you have the preservation of public health of this coast at heart. I believe you think I am trying to do honest effective work toward that same end. Your word will carry far more weight than mine. Is there anything you can do, say, or write, that will help me acquire the equipment that is absolutely essential for this work?"[30]

The bureau finally caved in and authorized the flexible hoses, and the *Omaha* was moved closer to the piers to facilitate the work.

The overall number of vessels fumigated or certified mounted to about 150 per week.[31] The *Sternberg* was back in operation, Wyman assigned two more commissioned officers to help out, and two competent local doctors were hired at a salary of $150 per month to patrol the wharves and make sure that all vessels complied with the docking rules. But MHS's workers still struggled to keep pace with the labor and the launches were wearing out.[32]

There were other problems. The temporary help hired for the fumigation were not reliable. They often quit, failed to show up for work, or were discharged for drunkenness and/or insubordination. The roster changed almost daily. Pay was low (a fumigator got $35 per month, a supervisor $50), and the work hard and dirty. In Dr. Hobdy's words, "The work was so heavy and the demand for pots so imperative that almost as soon as hatches were off my men swathed their heads in wet cloths, plunged into the fumes and brought off the pots and pans to take to some other vessel."[33] Pay on tugboats was higher and tugboat crews worked shorter hours.

It is no surprise that the feverish pace of the waterfront work, using toxic materials, would occasionally give rise to tragedy. In May 1908, after checking carefully that no one remained on board a French vessel, the fumigators lit the sulfur pots and closed the hatches. Not long after, a passing stevedore noted a distorted and panicky face pressed up against one of the portholes. Acting quickly, he broke the glass and hauled the gasping head through the hole into fresh air, while other bystanders stuffed gunnysacks around his neck to stop the outward flow of fumes. Rescuers charged onto the ship, opened the forecastle where the victim was, lifted him out, and rushed him, now unconscious, to the hospital. He regained enough consciousness to babble that he had a companion who was still on the ship. The news flashed back to the pier, but it was too late; the fumes had claimed the second man. Further inquiry disclosed that the two men were stowaways who had hidden in a chain locker below the forecastle, separated from it by a metal plate. They had been invisible during the pre-fumigation inspection.[34]

As winter arrived, storms harassed the teams, damaged more roofs at the station, and tore out part of the adjacent sea wall. Officers that worked on the boarding vessels, usually eating and sleeping on board, now worked from tugboats for boarding activities and did not have meals or sleeping quarters available. To get warm or come in from the rain they huddled in the old detention shed used by the Immigration Service, where the only space with heat was a 12 × 16–foot room already crowded with immigration personnel and other waterfront workers. The officers paid out of their own pockets for their food, although Washington finally remedied this after multiple requests from Hobdy.[35]

Eventually, the number of rats found after fumigations declined, though in many cases the number never declined to zero. Ferryboats and similar commuting craft that underwent fumigation every two weeks saw markedly lowered rat counts. Vessels that could not produce their certificate of disinfection or did not observe proper docking procedures simply had to undergo another disinfection.[36] Owners protested, particularly when dead rats were no longer found, but their complaints, whether directed to Washington or the state health department, went nowhere. Newspaper ridicule had grown and was ignored as well. Hobdy stressed to Wyman that all the money and time spent on fumigation would be wasted if a vessel were allowed to convey plague-infested rats upriver to new towns.[37] In the first five months, Hobdy's crews had fumigated about fifteen hundred outgoing vessels and burned almost 500,000 pounds of sulfur. In spite of this, he confided that he remained concerned that careless ship captains would carry plague upriver to new areas.[38] In October, in fact, three cases turned up in Seattle, suspected, though not proven, to have come from San Francisco.[39]

In February 1908, about six months after the rat fumigation began, Wyman asked about reducing fumigations since rat counts were consistently lower. The governor asked the same question. Hobdy again said no, noting that Wyman's figures were unreliable. Most counts that Wyman saw came from ship captains, who wanted less-frequent treatments, while counts carried out by Hobdy's men were higher. On the wharves, it was true that inspectors saw fewer rats, though Hobdy attributed this to the winter rains that drove rats indoors. And even though human cases had dropped off, the percentage of rats caught that were infected had actually increased from 0.5 percent to 1.5 percent, a tripling of the rate. Since this was an average figure, some areas showed higher rates.[40] Hobdy added that he would have felt personally responsible should plague spread to another port. The few cases in Seattle and the experience in Australia were no doubt on his mind. The fumigations continued.

As the battle against rats rolled on, the question was finally raised as to whether the species of rat was important in plague transmission. Were some rats more liable than others to transmit plague? An inquiry came from Wyman asking for a breakdown of rat types in San Francisco. Remarkably, no one knew what species were riding on sea vessels. Hobdy replied that he would investigate as soon as possible.[41] Studies eventually showed that three species predominated in the area: *Rattus rattus, Rattus norvegicus,* and *Rattus alexandrinus.*[42] *Rattus norvegicus* was the least common rodent found on ships, since it cannot nest in that environment. All types of rats carried fleas, the purveyors of plague.

Hobdy was under immense stress. In addition to the taxing fumigation work in the face of grumbling ship captains, vessels still arrived intermittently carrying smallpox victims. The quarantine of passengers and crews, sometimes in the hundreds, removed Hobdy from the fumigation efforts closer to shore. Seven instances of quarantine for smallpox drew him away from the rat-killing fumigations during the fiscal year ending June 30, 1908. In addition, in late December his young son developed pneumonia. The child's temperature soared to 105 degrees, accompanied by convulsions, adding sleepless nights to Hobdy's long days in an era before antibiotic remedies. Thankfully, by early February his son was recuperating. Hobdy mentioned the illness in a letter to a friend, but never in the official dispatches.[43]

The number of new plague cases in San Francisco eventually fell off, and the last case was recorded in February 1908. Overall, 159 people had been afflicted, with 77 deaths.[44] By this time, fumigators were finding far fewer rats on the outgoing ships, and on May 25, 1908, the frequency of fumigations was cut in half. Vessels receiving treatment every thirty days now waited sixty days, with proportionate reductions for vessels fumigated with less frequency.[45] The furious pace of fumigation had consumed a total of 620,000 pounds of sulfur. Finally, on October 21, 1908, the fumigation operations ceased.[46] Two days later the last rat in San Francisco known to be infected with plague was captured. The next 60,000 examined were free of disease.[47] About a million rats had been killed and thousands of fumigations carried out. Except for the three cases in Seattle, not a single case of plague turned up in the innumerable small landing sites dotting the rivers or along the coast, a remarkable achievement.

Plague and cholera continued to haunt various Asian and Latin American ports, however. The Angel Island Quarantine Station, though relieved of the frenzy of constant fumigations, was forced to remain on constant alert. Rats, previously neglected during ship inspections, were now the center of attention. In a similar manner, the inspection of passengers and crew focused particularly on signs of plague. Meanwhile, the station continued to grow and was reaching full size. And, at the same time, a new neighbor moved in: the Immigration Service.

CHAPTER NINE

Full Maturity and Immigration

As the second decade of the new century unfolded, the quarantine station continued to expand and develop. New structures gradually filled in the sloping area as funds became available, while older ones underwent repair at a slow—sometimes too slow—rate. By 1915 there were forty-one structures on the station. Thirty-five workers, including the medical officers and boat crews, staffed the facility.[1]

In 1912 funds arrived to build an improved roof on the original rough-hewn barracks built by the O&O Steamship Company as an emergency measure when the station first opened. The interior of the barracks underwent refurbishing during the next year. More widely spaced and more comfortable bunks replaced the tightly spaced ones. The quarantined passengers now used flush toilets instead of using a privy, and enjoyed the safer steam heat that substituted for space heaters. These barracks retained the nickname Chinese Barracks (buildings #18 and #19), while building #14 was the Japanese Barracks. Equipment for basic clinical testing, bacteriology, and animal inoculation served the laboratory needs. Two lazarettos for quarantinable diseases and a contagious disease hospital for other easily transmitted diseases, such as scarlet fever and mumps, stood ready. Miscellaneous buildings included a blacksmith's shop, a stable, a carpentry and machine shop, along with a laundry, greenhouse, pump house, power station, kitchens, and office space. The bathhouse for showering steerage passengers, the shed for the giant sterilizers, and a boathouse, all clustered near the pier, had been modernized as needed. Most of the other buildings served as living and dining quarters for the medical personnel, nurse, pharmacist, and various attendants. Similar accommodations were available for cabin and second-class passengers in quarantine (who were spared the barracks if at all possible).

Overall, in 1917 the station had facilities for 117 first-class, 29 second-class, and 477 steerage-class passengers (165 Japanese and 312 Chinese—the two groups were kept separate if possible). The few European steerage passengers who turned up were lodged in facilities for second-class passengers or sometimes remained on their ship.[2]

Maintenance was a constant problem, partly due to the salty air. Metal fixtures and pipes tended to corrode, paint peeled readily, and rugs grew moldy. These and other maintenance problems were persistent challenges. Damage from stormy weather, especially landslides, kept the personnel busy during slack times and intermittently strained the budget. In January 1914 another storm blew off a roof, scattered numerous shingles, knocked out glass windows, and toppled several trees. Heavy rains that followed caused an estimated 250 tons of dirt and rock to slip in a landslide, carrying freshwater and saltwater piping with it.[3] Intramural telephone lines also failed during heavier storms, at which time messages were delivered from building to building by hand, often up a steep hill.

Some aspects of station life were slow to advance. After havoc from another runaway horse, Hobdy pleaded for a truck, reassuring Wyman that it would soon pay for itself. In addition, he complained, horses smelled, and "from the sanitary standpoint they and the stable are an embarrassment."[4] A truck finally arrived—a Ford—in 1918, and the horses were gradually abandoned.[5] Purchasing, previously done by the station, was taken over by a new bureau of supply, which proved less efficient. Three newly ordered trucks arrived without carburetors, magnetos, batteries, or oil cups.[6] By the early 1920s, oil replaced coal as the power source for the electric street and house lighting, though electricity was only available at certain hours (no current after 11:30 P.M., for example). Coal, to the tune of eighteen tons a month, continued to provide power for most other functions, such as heating.[7]

Sewage disposal was an embarrassment for many years. The drainage pipes were too short and emptied onto the beach adjacent to Raccoon Strait. At low tide the effluent was unsightly and stank, and at high tide the current did not completely wash the sewage into the Bay.[8] Compounding the smell, the Army at one point repaired a utility road that ran around the station, using manure as a fill material for depressions in the surface. Between the road, the horses, and sewage on the beach the odors intensified and the fly population exploded.[9] Finally, in 1916 the sewerage pipes were extended to enter the Bay at a proper depth. Sewage still polluted the Bay, but less visibly.[10] Rats, too, shared the island, hiding under the older wooden, damp buildings. Trapping and poison helped but failed to eliminate them.[11] A few small blessings, though, included freedom from roaches and bedbugs and infrequent mosquitoes.

Freshwater continued to be scarce in the dry season. The existing well was not deep enough to compensate for variations in the amount of rain from year to year, and supplementary water was ferried in by boat. The station needed 6,000 to 10,000 gallons daily, depending on the season, and up to an extra 10,000 per day when quarantined passengers filled the barracks. Eventually, a well dug to 302 feet supplied thirty gallons a minute of water that was described as sweet and clear, in spite of being drawn from soil surrounded by saltwater.[12] The deeper well put the water problem to rest.

The staff on the island enjoyed advantages and disadvantages. Pay was low in comparison to similar work elsewhere. The officer in charge frequently solicited raises for the personnel, pointing out that the cost of living in San Francisco was 25 percent higher than other cities. At one point the chief engineer, who could only go home on Sundays, had received $80 a month for eleven years. Next door at the Immigration Station (paid through the US Department of Commerce and Labor), the engineers received $135 a month for an eight-hour day and could have their family at the station or go home to the city any night.[13] But pleading for raises generally was met with objections that money was tight. Most personnel hung on to their jobs rather than quit, probably for certain attractive benefits. The staff was free from layoffs in slack periods, they received free medical care through the MHS hospital system, worker's compensation for injuries (not a widespread practice at the time), and most received paid lodging. Meals were substantial and, on average, the attendant staff's duties entailed relatively little hard physical labor in comparison with comparable positions elsewhere.[14] Fumigation work, of course, was an exception.

It was probably not an ideal place for a head of family to work. Social interaction was limited. Schools or playgrounds for children were absent and the staff enjoyed limited amusements, though a tennis court had been installed. One officer with small children requested permission to reside in the city, but the request was discouraged by the officer in charge. Presence on the island was needed, the chief said, and furthermore, "This is probably the most pleasant quarantine reservation in the Service [MHS] and, with few exceptions, is the least isolated and inaccessible."[15] That may have been so, but San Francisco was an inviting city.

One year the station pharmacist committed suicide. The pharmacist actually did relatively little pharmaceutical work. His principal burden was non-pharmaceutical paperwork—compiling reports, keeping inventory records, and the like. Glover, the station chief at the time, speculated that the strain of extra end-of-the-year paperwork was a contributing factor.[16]

The crew on the boarding vessel *Argonaut* was an essential part of the team but did not reside on the island. They worked long hours, starting to board incoming ships at sunup and continuing to sundown, in fair weather and foul. By 1930 most ships had electric lights and could be inspected after sunset, adding to the hours of duty. The crew's pay was also on the low end of the scale and turnover was frequent. Like most sea vessels, the *Argonaut* hosted its complement of cockroaches, spurring one imaginative crewmember to devise an efficient trap: He took a tin can, not over three inches high, put a layer of molasses on the bottom and placed on top a metal disc with an opening in the center. The curious roach peeked through the opening, extended his antennae to the molasses below, liked the smell, and dropped inside where he was captured by the gluey syrup. "Over four hundred roaches were caught *each night for a month* by this method," concluded the report (italics added).[17]

Due to the nature of quarantine duties, the intensity of work varied tremendously. At times, hundreds of passengers could descend on the station, testing the limits of its abilities. At most other times, routine maintenance was the order of the day. It was a feast or famine, storm or millpond, state of affairs. In early January 1910, for example, the US Navy cruiser SS *Washington* arrived from Japan with 976 men on board, two of them with smallpox. Five others had already died of that disease, and three more eventually needed isolation and the rest were held in quarantine; 568 of the total filled the barracks and cabin-class rooms. The remainder slept in dining areas and wherever they could find a few feet of space. Due to the reduced dining space the enlistees ate on verandas around the Japanese Barracks, taking advantage of unseasonably warm weather. In the Japanese Barracks the toilets functioned poorly. Heavy usage clogged the sewerage lines and toilets elsewhere were also unpredictable, as were corroding showerheads in the cabin class baths. The freshwater supply ran out in the first two days and the enlistees took saltwater showers followed by a dousing with a bucket of freshwater. The commanding officer, Dr. Trotter, was surprised that the men remained cheerful and free of

complaints throughout the two weeks of confinement.[18] A similar overflow occurred ten years later when a crew of 510 sailors exposed to smallpox sat out the quarantine.[19]

In reality, the quarantine barracks lay empty most of the time, thanks
to the prevalence of early vaccination and medical screening abroad.[20]
The Surgeon General had posted more officers at foreign ports and established telegraphic connections with major Central and South American
ports.[21] During several years the station handled only one or two quarantines for smallpox and none for other diseases.[22] Occasional errors in
bills of health led to extra disinfections, but overall the system functioned
well.[23] Even after the Panama Canal opened in 1914, the increased traffic
from South America and faraway India generated no extra quarantines.

Maintaining such a large facility for only occasional use might have
appeared extravagant, but readiness for large passenger loads was essential. As stated in a PHMHS publication, "The actual problem which con-
fronts a quarantine officer is the maintenance of an institution during
long or short periods of practical nonuse at such a state of efficiency and
preparedness that he can on two hours' notice handle a passenger steamer,
perhaps a large one, infected with quarantinable disease."[24] Especially
challenging was maintaining morale during slack times. Periods of quarantine activity continued to decline, however, and officials began to consider whether the elaborate system might well be modified.

Another question troubled quarantine authorities: occasionally persons living in areas where cholera was active carried cholera bacilli in their
stool after recovery from illness or were carriers of the bacteria without
symptoms. What risk did they pose if allowed to go onshore, and should
such a carrier be detected and isolated? To be safe, MHS decided to culture
stool samples of all steerage-class passengers from China and Japan over
an approximately five-month period from October 1916 to February 1917.
The research was valuable, showing that 3,449 consecutive cultures for
Vibrio cholera were negative. Routine culturing was abandoned.[25] Further
research showed that carriage of cholera organisms was probably not
important in the spread of the disease.[26]

In 1910 the Immigration Service, after using the detention shed for
processing passengers for years, finally opened a new facility on the eastern end of Angel Island. The station was intended to be a major upgrade,
equipped with a hospital, laboratory, and dormitory facilities. But there
had been significant delays during construction and the work was barely

completed by the opening day. The press had been lauding the new station as a paradise with spacious facilities and a modern hospital and compared it to a summer resort or a first-class hotel. But Commissioner of Immigration Hart Hyatt North privately complained of the serious delays and inadequate size of the station.[27] When the PHMHS officer, Dr. Glover, made his initial visit, he found the station to be overcrowded, poorly designed, and lacking proper toilet facilities. The hospital was too small, was deficient in sanitary arrangements, and had no provision for patients with contagious diseases other than those available at the quarantine station. Wyman, during a visit, stated that the hospital provided fairly satisfactory facilities but it was "by no means as spacious as it should be for the character of immigration entering the port of San Francisco."[28] The whole station was deficient in freshwater, a deficiency not corrected until 1918, and the risk of fire was considered serious.[29] The PHMHS continued to supply medical officers to examine immigrants, and the medical officers also ran the hospital at the new Immigration Station. Medical examination and treatment of immigrants, as before, focused on the ability to work and avoid becoming a public charge.[30]

Many immigrants with active disease, including those with Class A problems like venereal disease and mild trachoma, were now able to receive treatment in the hospital by PHMHS physicians in hopes of a cure; if cured, they were generally allowed to enter the country. The detention shed became a relic of the past. Although the Immigration Station was busy and frequently dubbed the Ellis Island of the West, it saw only a modest number of immigrants compared to its cousin in New York.

As medical knowledge expanded, so did questions. Public Health Service[31] doctors, for example, became aware that many immigrants carried parasites in their intestinal tract. Did carriers of various parasites pose a health risk to the immigrant? And what was the risk that the parasite would become disseminated in the local environment? In particular, what should be done with those harboring hookworm, a common parasitic infection of the rural poor, spread primarily by skin contact with soil contaminated with fecal matter? After the takeover of Puerto Rico in the Spanish-American War, hookworms had been pinpointed, along with a poor diet, as the cause of anemia, weakness, and swollen bellies prevalent in the local population.[32] Similar findings turned up in the rural American south. Treatment, supplemented with a healthy diet and iron, restored normal vigor and strength to those afflicted.[33]

The revised *Book of Instructions for the Medical Inspection of Aliens,* published in 1910, the year the Immigration Station opened, put hookworm (also called *uncinariasis*) in the Class A category of loathsome and contagious diseases, a category requiring deportation.[34] It was believed that hookworm infection, if untreated, would hamper a person's ability to earn a livelihood. Fortunately, hookworm infestation was a treatable condition and, despite being in Class A, only a small percentage of carriers were deported, the rest allowed in after treatment.[35] An exception was the rejection of a large number of South Asians in 1911.[36]

Screening and treatment for parasite infestation were labor-intensive. The stool sample had to be collected, processed, and examined under a microscope. If hookworm eggs came into view the patient underwent a treatment that might last several days (thymol, in varying doses, was most frequently used). The laborious process soon overwhelmed the hospital facilities, causing serious delays. For example, during the fiscal year 1911–12 the hospital admitted 998 patients with hookworm, of whom 958 were discharged as recovered.[37] To help out, the hospital at the quarantine station handled some of the excess laboratory processing.[38]

To reduce the workload, in 1913 the Immigration Service required that immigrants obtain a certificate testifying that they were free of hookworm before arrival in California.[39] This had limited success.[40] Finally, in 1917 hookworm infection was reclassified to Class B, and no longer a reason for deportation if treated.[41] Many immigrants were understandably embarrassed or felt degraded by undergoing examinations in the nude and submitting stool samples, procedures they were unaccustomed to.[42]

Other parasites, whose natural history was uncertain at the time, were found in smaller numbers of immigrants. Filaria (parasites found swimming in the blood stream) and amoebas (a cause of lower intestinal disease) could result in deportation. One that especially aroused the anger of the Chinese Six Companies was the Chinese liver fluke, *Clonorchis sinensis,* a worm that infests the liver and whose eggs are discharged into the intestinal tract. Its biology was virtually unknown when first seen by the Public Health Service doctors. The worm had received no mention in the 1910 *Book of Instructions.* In 1917 the liver fluke was placed in Category A, meaning deportation, until more research was done to evaluate the clinical course of patients afflicted with it and to determine whether eggs discharged into sewage could implant the parasite permanently in the environment. Ten years later, studies concluded that, though no effective treatment had been found, the infestation proved to be indolent in most cases and was not liable to spread in the United States. It was downgraded to category C.[43] The Public Health Service medical officers were not involved in evaluating the status of an immigrant beyond the physical and laboratory examinations carried out, though their diagnoses were usually determinant.

In 1917 a new immigration bill required all immigrants and all alien (non-US citizen) ship crews, regardless of whether they planned to go onshore or not, to be inspected by *two* medical officers.[44] The extra burden on the quarantine station's medical inspectors created new bottlenecks for ship captains. Among ship crews, venereal disease was the main problem keeping the Public Health Service doctors busy.[45]

A combination of overcrowding and poor maintenance led to deterioration of the Immigration Station. Lack of cleanliness, rude treatment of immigrants, and poor food were major problems. In 1922 the commissioner general of immigration, after an inspection, commented, "Angel Island has the worst immigration station I have ever visited. The plant has nothing to commend it. It is made up of a conglomeration of buildings which are nothing but fire traps. They are illy [*sic*] arranged and inconvenient. The sanitary arrangements are awful."[46] He suggested a new facility on the mainland, though that would not come to pass until 1940 after a fire destroyed most of the buildings.

By 1914 Europe was at war. Almost simultaneously, the Panama Canal opened, allowing sea traffic from eastern ports to pass to California. The following year, San Francisco hosted the Panama–Pacific International Exposition, built to celebrate the opening of the Canal and to showcase San Francisco's stunning recovery from the devastating earthquake. Built on the northern shore of the city, the massive enterprise included an artificial lake; the huge French Pavilion (a replica of the Palais de la Légion d'Honneur in Paris, later to be reproduced as the Palace of the Legion of Honor Museum); a Tower of Jewels, glittering with 100,000 cut-glass Novagems; the Bernard Maybeck–designed Palace of Fine Arts; a Japanese tea house; the famous Liberty Bell, brought out from Philadelphia; and many other installations and amusements.[47] Yacht and motorboat racing, along with aquatic displays, provided entertainment on the Bay's waters. Brilliant electric lighting lit up the sky at night, surely a splendid sight for those at the quarantine station who ventured up the hill for a view. The beauty and gaiety of the Exposition provided a counterpoint to the ugly war in Europe.

The European conflict did not immediately affect activities at the station since America was still neutral. In 1917 activity fell more dramatically as the United States became a belligerent and ship traffic diminished. In 1918 the station temporarily housed about 450 interned Germans, and the following year a group of American troops serving in the American Expeditionary Force in Russia returned from Siberia to be deloused. They were stripped and bathed with a mixture of soap and gasoline, while their clothes went through the giant steam sterilizers.[48]

In the waning months of the war another enemy struck, one that did not use bullets and cannons but infiltrated silently: influenza. The massive influenza epidemic reached San Francisco in September of 1918, about two months before the end of the Great War.[49] By mid-October, close to four hundred people a day were stricken, many of them gasping their last breaths. A peak attack rate of 2,005 cases in one day was reached on October 25.[50]

Theaters, movie houses, dance halls, and other public gathering spots were closed. Clergy sometimes held outdoor services but more often cancelled church services and encouraged their parishioners to pray at home. Schools shut down. Wearing masks in public, recommended at first, became mandatory. The governor and the mayor, using slogans from the war, declared that it was a patriotic duty to wear a mask. Those found without them were fined and some were jailed. One day, in a surprise raid on downtown hotels, about one hundred maskless guests were arrested.[51] On another day Mayor James Rolph was fined $50 by his own police chief for being in public without a mask. Signs reading, "Influenza—wear your mask and save your life," were visible everywhere, and the Red Cross set up stands to sell the masks.

Hospitals filled up quickly and were soon overwhelmed. The San Francisco General Hospital sent all its pre-epidemic patients home or to other care sites and made its five hundred beds available for influenza cases. At the Civic Center a Red Cross administration building became a three-hundred-bed hospital, and several open-air hospitals sprouted up.[52] Letterman Hospital, on the Presidio Army base, doubled its capacity from 1,100 beds to 2,200 to handle the load.[53] Nurses were in short supply, many of them already victims, and teachers were recruited to help with the nursing care of children. Thousands of residents lined up to receive a vaccine, though the vaccine, made from bacteria incorrectly thought to be the cause of influenza pneumonia, was ineffective. A dip in new cases in late November led to a relaxation of the isolation rules. Theaters, then schools, opened up and masks stayed in drawers. Then a resurgence of cases in January 1919 brought back a reinforcement of previous regulations. Only as spring arrived did the epidemic subside and the population began to throw away the masks and make their way back to schools, churches, and entertainments. Overall, nearly 45,000 people in San Francisco came down with influenza, over 3,000 of whom perished.[54]

The quarantine station played only a small role in the flu epidemic. More than a hundred cadets from a nearby naval training ship stayed in quarantine at the station after an outbreak, and the station's hospital staff cared for overflow patients from the MHS Hospital in San Francisco.[55] Several station personnel were felled by the virus, though none died from it.[56]

At the end of the second decade of the twentieth century, the Public Health Service finally assumed control of all local quarantine stations around the country. A unified, national system was now in place under the aegis of the Public Health Service.[57] The San Francisco Quarantine Station was at peak size. In the following decades quarantine activity diminished— gradually at first, then more rapidly. Improved vaccination rates and more complete knowledge of the modes of transmission of cholera, plague, and yellow fever had reduced the risks of imported epidemic disease. The practice of placing quarantine stations in remote locations, such as Angel Island, was undergoing review. The old belief that contagious diseases were spread through the air, requiring remote sites for quarantining passengers, had faded. Research had revealed that plague, yellow fever, and typhus are all transmitted by an insect vector. Cholera is transmitted through contaminated water and food, not air. And smallpox, the only quarantinable disease transmitted by the respiratory route, finds its way from host to host at relatively short distances. Given the improved knowledge of disease transmission, isolation on islands no longer made sense, and the location on Angel Island underwent reevaluation. "Not only is the maintenance of the station unnecessarily burdensome, but the isolation works a hardship alike on officers and employees at the station," wrote Rupert Blue, who was by then surgeon general, in 1918. He suggested that the quarantine station be moved from Angel Island to the north shore of San Francisco.[58]

Another concept was under reevaluation. For years the quarantine services had been disinfecting ships, clothing, luggage, and passengers as a means of halting disease at the waterfront. At the onset, the idea was to eliminate germs, realized as the purveyors of disease. Over time, however, with the new discoveries mentioned above, the practice of disinfecting an entire ship seemed unnecessary. By 1910 it was clear that plague control rested on rat control, that smallpox prevention depended on isolation of cases and vaccination, that cholera prevention was achieved through clean food and water supplies, that yellow fever was prevented by mosquito control, and typhus was curtailed by eliminating lice. In 1912 Leland E. Cofer, chief of the division of quarantine, a new division created in the expanding Public Health Service, wrote a pamphlet entitled, *A Word to Ship Captains about Quarantine*. He laid out the above principles and made it clear that other measures were unimportant in controlling epidemic disease.[59] Ship disinfection, in the sense in which it was formerly used, seemed to have little practical value, except for the use of fumigation to control rats and cockroaches, and it died out. Disinfection of mail, once a routine practice, had been discontinued earlier.

The threat of plague, San Francisco's main quarantine concern by this time, did not go away. The disease flared up intermittently in Asia and in coastal cities in South America. Frequent ship fumigations lowered the rat populations significantly but did not eliminate them. Rats from infected ports still hitched a ride on vessels bound for San Francisco. Quarantine stations in other US ports were also uneasy about plague. Plague did, in fact, return to the United States, making an unwelcome appearance in New Orleans in 1916. New Orleans, the city that had confronted yellow fever and created a ship cleansing technique to deal with it, now faced plague and plague-infested rats. Perhaps it is fitting that the birthplace of the ship disinfection techniques adopted at Angel Island was also the birthplace of a new technique for plague prevention: cyanide fumigation. The southern port's new weapon had major implications for rat control on San Francisco Bay.

CHAPTER TEN

The Cyanide Era

EVENTS ABROAD COMBINED TO heighten anxiety about the reintroduction of plague into San Francisco, indeed to all American ports. China was in tumult. As the Qing dynasty teetered and finally collapsed in the revolution of 1911, the new government functioned erratically at best. The ensuing political turmoil, aggravated by uprisings, poorly controlled warlords, and general disorganization, was disruptive. In 1910–11 China suffered the worst plague epidemic since the catastrophic plague event in India not long before, with the later epidemic claiming about 60,000 lives.[1] Though the primary focus was in Manchuria and did not materially affect the more southern ports, California felt threatened. Other countries voiced similar fears, forcing the Chinese government to assign a higher priority to public health policies. In the wake of the Manchurian epidemic, for example, the government created the Manchurian Plague Prevention Service specifically to interact with other powers.[2]

The Public Health Service had stationed health officers in Amoy, Hong Kong, Kobe, Nagasaki, Shanghai, and Yokohama. By 1910–11 those health officers reported improving conditions in the respective ports, with fewer cases of plague and smallpox, fewer rats, and overall enhancement in the cleansing of departing ships.[3] Rodent plague simmered below the surface, however, and additional human cases continued to appear in Asian ports. South American ports saw similar troubles, as Rupert Blue reported after a fact-finding tour: "As regards plague, it would be wise...to declare the entire coast of Chile infected," he wrote in 1910.[4] Many other ports were similarly affected. In the San Francisco Bay, it was still easy to find rats on incoming ships, even those from Honolulu, and any rat was a potential plague carrier.[5]

Wyman, frustrated by the continued presence of rats on incoming ships, decided to mount a frontal attack, initiating a campaign that he dubbed rat quarantine.[6] In October 1910 he issued new regulations, stipulating that ships "shall have such measures taken as will free them from rats not less than every six months." [7] Wyman sent a formal order to the Angel Island station the following April, ordering ships from plague-infested ports to be fumigated every six months specifically to kill rats. The fumigations could be carried out at San Francisco or at the originating port provided there was a Public Health and Marine Hospital Service (PHMHS) officer on hand to supervise it, the choice being up to the captain's convenience. After each fumigation, in order to assay the effectiveness of the program, rats had to be counted. [8] Washing of decks and cabin walls had been pretty well abandoned by this time, a bow to the evidence that such washing was not helpful. This trend was reinforced when public health workers found that washing walls in houses of individuals infected with contagious diseases did not affect further spread. [9]

The new fumigation policy specifically included upper-level cabins, galleys, and other compartments. Fumigation in holds had driven rats from their cavernous homes to cozier refuges higher up, where they found warmth and often food. Since sulfur dioxide could damage or alter certain materials, including clothing, the crewmembers removed their clothing and personal effects before the fumigation began, then waited for several hours after fumigation to return them. They also had to repaint discolored walls and repolish tarnished metal at intervals, due to the effects of the sulfur. But the efforts paid off. In the year ending June 30, 1912, 3,811 rats from 144 vessels met their death. Most of those rats had been found in cabins, storerooms, and other upper-level spaces rather than holds. [10] Even fumigation every six months was not enough for ships from some ports—Hong Kong, for instance, on which rat counts remained high. Wyman authorized those ships to be fumigated as often as needed. [11]

Though the rat quarantine was in effect at all US coastal quarantine stations, at least one plague-ridden rat slipped ashore, this time in New Orleans. The rat was discovered in 1912, but it was an isolated finding and no other infected rats were found among thousands examined. Two uneventful years passed until a pair of workers in a horse stable complained of weakness, chills, rising temperatures, and swollen, painful lymph glands. The laboratory diagnosed the illness as plague after examining an aspirate from a swollen gland. One of the men perished. His death was followed by a full outbreak of plague that took a little more than ten years to fully eradicate. [12]

Foreign countries, fearing for their own ports, insisted that ships leaving New Orleans be treated for rats. The quarantine service instituted sulfur dioxide fumigation of all departing ships, just as in San Francisco several years earlier, then switched to the use of carbon monoxide. The Cuban government, however, required that ships from New Orleans be fumigated with cyanide before entering Cuban ports. They reasoned that cyanide, by killing off rats and their fleas, was preferable to carbon monoxide that killed only rats.[13]

Cyanide fumigation, in the form of hydrocyanic acid gas, had been around for some time, though not on ships. As early as the 1880s, California citrus growers had found it indispensable for protecting their trees from insect damage. The growers draped the trees with a covering tent, into which the hydrocyanic acid gas was released and retained for a period of time.[14] The success of the method, and the resistance of citrus rinds to penetration of the poison, made it a popular insecticide. In 1921, according to a major manufacturer, the American Cyanamid Company, about one-third of the 20 million citrus trees in California were fumigated this way, the remaining trees contributing little to the total crop. Two and one-half million yards of cloth were needed just for the tentage.[15]

The PHMHS had in fact approved hydrocyanic acid gas as a fumigant in 1910, but fear of its inherent danger stalled its use.[16] Quarantine officials in Puerto Rico appear to have been the first to use it, in 1912, to avoid damage to Canary Island vegetables from sulfur fumigation. No harm came to the vegetables or to those who ate them.[17] Hydrocyanic acid gas is highly toxic, not only to insects and rodents, but also to humans. Being odorless and colorless, it is also undetectable, rendering it especially dangerous to use. Inhaling small amounts will ensure a quick death, as was shown by its repeated use in concentration camps during World War II.

New Orleans acceded to Havana's demands and adopted cyanide fumigation.[18] This fumigation technique offered advantages in spite of the danger: It worked rapidly. It diffused into nooks and crannies in cargo holds that were not reached easily by sulfur dioxide. It efficiently penetrated materials such as mattresses, pillows, blankets, and the like. Virtually all materials were safe from harm and residual odor, which was certainly not the case with sulfur dioxide. It eliminated the frightening need to burn sulfur on oil tankers. Cyanide gas also decimated cockroaches and bedbugs, both constant and unwelcome companions on ships, that were not fully destroyed by sulfur. Some ship captains used cyanide for that purpose alone.

Cyanide's lethal effect, though, was a mixed blessing. Because the gas could not be seen or smelled, a fumigator who inadvertently inhaled the undetectable vapors risked a rapid death. Careless application techniques could cost lives, and to maximize safety the Public Health Service issued strict guidelines.[19]

The gas itself was generated by dropping a small quantity of potassium or sodium cyanide, wrapped in cheesecloth-like material, into a container of diluted sulfuric acid. The odorless fumes rose soon after. In preparation for cyanide fumigation, all crew and passengers were removed from the ship and accounted for on a roster, and the captain or first officer signed a form attesting to this. The fumigating crew worked out a specific route that ensured a single path through the ship with no retracing of steps. They then placed a bucket of sulfuric acid in each compartment and closed all relevant hatches and portholes. When all was in place, the fumigators walked the prearranged course, entering each compartment to drop a packet of cyanide into the sulfuric acid bucket, then scurrying out of the compartment and closing the door to seal in the emerging vapors. To fumigate sizable holds the crew lowered a large barrel of sulfuric acid into the space. A small bucket containing the cyanide packet was mounted on a swivel over each barrel. After evacuating the hold, the crew on deck pulled on a rope running from the bottom of the mounted bucket to the hatch above, tipping the bucket and allowing the cyanide to slide into the waiting barrel of sulfuric acid. The hatch was then sealed, permitting the gas to do its work.

The cyanide gas remained at least one hour in compartments and longer in holds when cargo was present. After opening the doors and hatches, the crew allowed at least fifteen minutes for compartments and one hour for holds to clear the fumes (later extended to longer periods). The use of fans was recommended to facilitate airing out. Then the crew introduced a small animal, a guinea pig or mouse, kept in a wire cage, into the compartment. If it remained healthy, the area was safe to enter. The officer in charge made any final decisions about entering.[20] When the Navy tested the procedure, personnel carried, but did not use, oxygen respirators when opening the compartments.[21] Initially, the Public Health Service did not use any protective gear.

At San Francisco the cyanide method was first tried in the spring of 1913, on tankers. As mentioned earlier, tankers tied up to the *Omaha* for fumigation with sulfur dioxide pumped through a hose. In windy weather ships rolled and risked damage, delays, and extra expense if the tanker hull bruised the *Omaha* too forcefully. When tanker captains heard about the new cyanide method, they requested it in lieu of sulfur.[22]

Meanwhile, in February 1913, in response to heightened plague risks from abroad, the surgeon general issued supplementary orders. All vessels from ports in Africa, South America, Asia (including the Philippines), and the West Indies (except Puerto Rico) were to be fumigated for rats on arrival at US ports, regardless of prior inspections.[23] The extra burden, using the time-consuming sulfur fumigation, overwhelmed the station, pulling men from important other duties.[24] The plague team onshore in San Francisco that was still actively hunting, killing, and examining rats since the 1907 outbreak, helped out by collecting dead rats from fumigated vessels for examination and by patrolling the waterfront. In spite of the help, the station's personnel could not keep up with the increased load.[25]

Cargo vessels lingered at anchor or at docks, putting up with longer and more frequent delays. Their captains grew impatient and soon requested the new cyanide method to replace the cumbersome sulfur fumigations. Wyman and his quarantine service generally tried to accommodate shipping interests as long as public safety was not compromised. After waiting to ensure that the safety of cyanide matched its efficiency, Wyman officially sanctioned its broader use in mid-February 1916, under certain conditions.[26] All work must be done under the strict supervision of the quarantine service and the captain or first officer must sign a form certifying that all persons were off the ship and accounted for before any fumigation.[27] Due to the high cost of cyanide, the station agreed to pay only for the amount used to fumigate compartments, putting the shipping companies on the hook for the quantities used in holds. The ship owners gladly accepted, seeing the time saved as being well worth it.[28] As a side benefit, the method eliminated millions of cockroaches. According to one report, "It is not unusual to kill approximately 20,000 to 50,000 in a forecastle [crews' quarters], while more than 20,000 have been taken from a single small stateroom."[29]

Adverse events from cyanide were few. Occasional fumigators became ill from reentering compartments earlier than the stipulated time, prompting further precautions. "Danger—Keep Out" posters appeared on compartment doors, times until reentry were extended to allow more vapors to escape, and fumigation at night was forbidden. As will be evident, it is probable that fumigators did not always introduce caged rodents before reentering compartments, which was an essential safety precaution.

By the end of June of 1916, 72 vessels had been processed with cyanide gas in San Francisco, consuming 4,404 pounds of cyanide.[30] An unexpected surprise was that vessels previously fumigated with sulfur dioxide suddenly yielded hundreds of dead rats, making it clear that the old sulfur dioxide fumigations were not as effective as thought. Experience quickly showed that cyanide fumes penetrated well into poorly aerated corners and through semiporous materials, and they killed faster. A second cyanide fumigation yielded scanty rat counts, confirming again the superiority of the method.[31] Rat populations could be large. The highest count recorded that year was on a Mexican ship where 262 rats met their death. The Japanese ship SS *Persia Maru* harbored 259 rats, 52 of them recovered in two of its lifeboats. By 1920 almost five hundred vessels annually were being doused with cyanide.[32] At one point the combined use of cyanide for ship fumigation in the citrus industry and in the mining industry (where it was used in the separation of gold from ore), led to a national shortage. A small supply, located in Oakland, bought enough time for the quarantine crew to ride out the crisis.[33]

By common agreement, shipping companies provided their own fumigators, usually recruited from local stevedores. The Public Health Service supervised the work—deciding where to fumigate, making sure proper doses were used, and ensuring that all materials were handled properly. Ominously, reported the station chief, though no fatalities had occurred, "several sailors have been overcome by the gas and removed from compartments after fumigation."[34] Even close supervision could not remove all the risk, especially since the fumigators were not organized as professionally trained teams.

In October 1916 the Japanese fumigating crew of the *Tokiwa Mura* returned to their ship after a fumigation and found a man slumped over a pile of coal, lifeless. The ship's doctor and another crewmember, charging in to help him, almost lost their own lives.[35] The fumigation had apparently gone well, according to the station chief, W. A. Korn. On the other hand, a coroner's inquest concluded, "Death resulted from carelessness of the officers of the ship in not following the instructions given by the U.S. Quarantine Officers." The inquest recommended that further fumigations be done under the complete supervision of qualified Federal officers and that instructions for the ship be issued in language that the involved personnel could readily understand.[36] Details were not given but, presumably, the crewmember was not present and accounted for during the fumigation.

New rules called again for placement of a small, caged rodent into an aired room to test for residual gas before human entry. The use of mechanical ventilators was again recommended.[37] Guards were posted at strategic points.[38]

The very next month, on the Norwegian ship SS *Roald Amundsen*, hatches had been open for three hours after fumigation, a time well beyond the half hour stipulated in the instructions. A man lowered deep into the hold signaled frantically for help. Knowing that seconds counted, the crew on deck rapidly lowered others to retrieve him. They reached their colleague just in time to save him, though they too were sickened in the process. After reaching the deck again, the gasping crew noticed that one of their members was missing. More men plunged into the hold, only to find their mate already overcome and lifeless. All the fumigation precautions, including the timing of reentry, had apparently been observed.[39] At the coroner's inquest, however, a jury of seven concluded that the death was "largely due to the carelessness of the quarantine officials." They claimed that the instructions were written in poorly legible English. A press account did not add much, except that no animal had been introduced into the hold before entering, a breach in protocol.[40]

Further safety measures were implemented. Once again, the rules called for the introduction of small, caged rodents into rooms before reentry. The Division of Quarantine in Washington preferred rats to guinea pigs; they survived exposure more easily, allowing them to be used multiple times, thereby saving money.[41] The use of fans to air out spaces more rapidly became mandatory. Later, in 1920, gas masks were placed on board each ship being fumigated. Wearing them during fumigation was rejected, however, on the grounds that it might lead to carelessness. In Washington, a search was under way to find a substance to mix with the cyanide to color the air if toxic levels of gas were reached. The search was not successful.[42]

Two years passed without mishaps, then tragedy struck again, this time on a larger scale. The SS *Nanking*, owned by the China Mail Steamship Company, docked in September 1919, at a time when the stevedores were on strike. The ship's captain hired unskilled Mexican labor to unload the ship, following which the vessel underwent cyanide fumigation per protocol. After opening hatches and doors for aeration, a Public Health Service officer entered the forward steerage area and found three men, all lifeless. The three were Mexican, identified as temporary dock laborers, and two of them were on the payroll of the ship. The best guess was that the three had secreted themselves on board sometime between the inspection and the fumigation, probably as stowaways. An inquest provided no further insight and the deaths were ruled "accidental suffocation."[43]

Would these tragedies have occurred if a more professional crew had served as fumigators? No, stated the Owl Fumigating Company from Azusa, California. The recently organized company, hoping to secure a fumigation contract that promised to avoid disasters, approached the quarantine station commander. They offered to provide a thoroughly trained crew of fumigators that would work under the supervision of the Angel Island officers. The trained, permanent, crew would be less prone to errors than crews hastily hired by captains on the spot.[44] The Owl Company had also developed an apparatus for spraying liquid hydrocyanic acid that vaporized rapidly into gas, thus eliminating the cumbersome sulfuric acid bucket routine. The station chief declined the offer, mainly because the spray apparatus was deemed unsatisfactory. The company then renamed itself the Cyanide Fumigation Company and offered the same package deal to ships desiring fumigation not required by quarantine regulations. Captains signed up readily, partly as a way to eliminate cockroaches and bedbugs.

In time, the Angel Island officers decided that the spray apparatus functioned well and that the fumigation team worked professionally. The use of steady, trained labor in place of ad hoc stevedores was an advantage and saved money. The station chief at the time, Friench Simpson, with Wyman's approval, agreed to the method, as long as it was carried out under quarantine service supervision. Delighted ship owners, who no longer had to buy the chemicals and find labor, readily signed up for the service.[45]

The dangerous fumigations continued. Overall, in fiscal year 1920, 484 vessels out of a total of 610 inspected were doused with cyanide, consuming in the process almost 37,000 pounds of sodium cyanide.[46] The crews found fewer rats, attributing this to the high rate of cyanide fumigation (about 80 percent of vessels) and rat-proofing measures instituted by shipowners.[47] By 1922 rats were being recovered from only about 50 percent of vessels fumigated. Still, 2,896 rats were killed, almost all sent to the still-maintained Public Health Service plague laboratory in San Francisco. None carried any plague bacilli.[48]

But another tragic death, this time in Boston, unnerved the authorities in Washington. As a result, the Public Health Service assumed control

over the entire fumigation process, using their own supplies and personnel. The new policy was instituted nationwide and started on September 1,
1921.[49] For the San Francisco station, where more than five hundred vessels
per year received the cyanide treatment, this meant a substantial increase
in personnel and equipment. The Harbor Commission constructed a
new building on Meiggs' Wharf to house the extra fumigating equipment, while the quarantine station started hiring its own fumigation
crews.[50] The Cyanide Fumigation Company, however, was livid. In spite
of admirable work and no deaths, their contracts with shippers became
null and void after about one month's notice.[51] The company protested
vehemently, but without success. The Public Health Service was able, however, to fumigate ships at cost, providing another saving to ship owners.

The goal of the new policy was to improve safety, or so it was thought.
But tragedy proved hard to avoid. In December 1921, the fourth month
of the new policy, a passenger was found dead after fumigation of the
SS *Seiyo Maru*. Fellow passengers had seen him acting strangely during
the voyage, thinking he looked depressed. He was on the dock during the
fumigation, then disappeared. The final opinion was that the passenger
had hopped on board undetected when the ship deck sank to dock level
at low tide and had surreptitiously gone below to his fate.[52]

More tragedy was to follow. The following year, on February 28,
a crewmember collapsed after entering the hold of the British Ship
SS *Tahiti* and a second man, rushing to save him, paid with his own life
after inhaling the odorless fumes. Three others were hospitalized after
heroic rescue efforts. The *Tahiti* had been fumigated a few times previously at San Francisco without any difficulty.[53] The ship's hold was a
refrigerated area, and it was thought that the cold temperature (near freez-
ing) had kept the cooled gas sequestered near the bottom, thereby not
harming the inspector after aeration. As the hold warmed up the odorless cyanide gas presumably expanded and passed into the lungs of the
crewmember approaching from above. A coroner's inquest did not turn
up any other information, concluding that "the fumigating inspector was
negligent in his inspection," without further details.[54] The jury recommended that a specially trained and equipped rescue unit be available
for future emergencies. Friench Simpson's successor, Assistant Surgeon
General R. H. Creel, reviewing the case later, wrote that he was dubious
that an inspector had actually entered the refrigeration hold before allowing others in.[55]

Cyanide was abandoned once more, and sulfur dioxide fumigations restarted. The ship owners were unhappy, sending letters asking for resumption of cyanide fumigation. One of them, by the agents for the *Tahiti*, ended its plea with, "Although it was our steamer *Tahiti* where the unfortunate accident recently happened, we are quite satisfied to continue the use of cyanide in the future. We feel sure that in the hands of your department the likelihood of accidents from cyanide gas is not nearly as great as from a good deal of the work done in loading and unloading ships, let alone the other accidents to be met with in the calling of ship owning."[56] The medical director for plague suppressive measures in San Francisco (still functioning after the 1907 outbreak), J. G. Perry, weighed in, saying that cyanide was by far the best method of fumigation and, with additional safeguards, the risks would be sufficiently low.[57]

The surgeon general, faced with conflicting opinions, appointed a committee to study the problem, after which he yielded and gave permission in August to again resume cyanide fumigation. Power ventilators became mandatory and inspectors were required to carry (but not to wear) new gas masks as they tested the safety of reentering areas.[58] (Wearing the masks was still discouraged because it might lead to neglect of other safety measures.) And at least two people must inspect all compartments and holds and, once again, were to introduce a rat into compartments and holds before reentry. Emergency call numbers were posted.[59]

Reversion to cyanide fumigation pleased ship owners but proved catastrophic for the station. Less than a month later, five men died and another almost died during a single fumigation on the SS *Shinyo Maru*, a ship that the crew had fumigated once before. A full account of what happened never emerged since all five workers, the only first-hand witnesses, had perished. It appeared, though, that after noticing something amiss with a fumigator on a forward deck the other fumigators rushed to his rescue only to be overcome themselves by the poisonous vapors. Two nearby men on shore rushed to the ship and managed to pull one faltering rescuer to safety. Firefighters from a nearby fireboat also charged in but were too late to save any more. Several firefighters, in spite of wearing masks, were sickened but survived.[60]

The station chief, Friench Simpson, in a letter to the surgeon general, speculated that when placing the cyanide packets in the sulfuric acid containers (the spray apparatus had been abandoned) in the compartments something had gone wrong, perhaps a door not fully closed or a delay in the fumigator leaving the room. In addition, a strong wind was blowing in from the bow, which might have contributed to the disaster.[61]

Simpson offered more safety recommendations but he pessimistically admitted that "it cannot be hoped that there will be no fatalities since, in my opinion, deaths will inevitably occur as long as cyanide is used."[62] Simpson's successor, R. H. Creel, who had been stationed in New Orleans when cyanide was first introduced, reviewed the case and had little to add, though he sensed some laxity in carrying out the precautions.[63] He noted that the fumigating crews were small and overworked, and that their numbers were often supplemented with incompletely trained day labor.[64] The move from the professional crew of the Cyanide Fumigation Company to the crews hired and trained by the quarantine station had not been a success. Creel also tested some of the gas masks (a type known as the Burrell mask) and found that they did not fit the contour of the face well.[65]

At that point all cyanide fumigation was again suspended.[66] The human toll was truly excessive. From now on, tankers passed through without any fumigation at all and cargo ships were fumigated with sulfur dioxide or, if only part of their cargo was unloaded in San Francisco, sent on for terminal fumigation at a future port. If cyanide for rat killing was to continue, a safer approach was imperative.[67]

The Public Health Service had, in fact, called on the Army's Chemical Warfare Department for help. The chemists assigned to the task eventually came up with another agent that seemed to fulfill requirements.[68] It was called cyanogen chloride, and was a mixture of hydrocyanic acid gas, sodium chlorate, and hydrochloric acid, the latter two ingredients added as tearing agents, effectively turning the mixture into a tear gas. The irritation to the eyes warned a fumigator when significant gas levels were present. After some trial runs with the new mixture, the Public Health Service authorized the resumption of cyanide fumigation, not long after the *Shinyo Maru* incident.

Orders for the new agent went out by the end of the year, but since the station could no longer purchase directly, the order went through the Bureau of Supply. The first order was apparently ignored, and a second order, issued in late December, was filled but sent by ship through the Panama Canal rather than by rail freight, delaying its arrival until February 1923.[69]

The irritant effect of the new cyanogen chloride made one thing clear: many gas masks did not fit well, and better ones were obtained.[70]

The tearing additive probably saved one life—a stowaway on a ship in Baltimore was forced out of his hiding place in a rope locker when the gas stung his eyes. He survived.[71] The tearing effect irritated rats as much as humans, causing them to burrow deeper into small spaces or padding, but the cyanide reached them, nonetheless. Ship captains were happy again because the operation saved time, but also because cyanide fumigation destroyed cockroaches and other vermin in addition to rats.[72] Introducing rats into a room before entering no longer seemed necessary as the stinging and tearing felt by inspectors provided a sufficient warning.[73] It finally ceased.

The fumigators' work was still difficult and dangerous, and the pay quite modest. Turnover was high and suitable applicants hard to find. Furthermore, new rules had placed hiring in the hands of the local Civil Service Agency. Creel, station chief at the time (1923), complained that applicants were arriving who had no prior experience and who had passed an examination quiz that was "comparable to the test given at Ellis Island for determining feeble-mindedness."[74] Others had disabilities not suitable for the hazardous work, and Creel fired one for stealing liquor from a ship that he was fumigating.[75] Regardless, fumigation went on, and without fatalities.

Easier and safer methods continued to be developed. Improved spray cans finally replaced the practice of dropping cyanide into buckets of sulfuric acid. Another innovation was Zyklon-B, hydrocyanic acid absorbed into diatomaceous earth (a powdery substance formed from fossilized algae), an innovation introduced in late 1926. For safety, chloropicrin was added as an eye irritant. It was packaged as a powder to be sprinkled into holds or compartments where it vaporized after application. The residual cyanide-free powder was swept up and tossed overboard. Less equipment and fewer personnel were required to apply it, making it cheaper and more efficient.[76] Zyklon-B is the form of cyanide later used in German concentration camps. It showed some tendency to flammability, requiring care on hot days, and a few cockroaches resisted its effects because of the dilution with the tearing agent. The Angel Island station used both methods—the spray and the powder. The principal advance, though, had been the addition of tearing agents to the cyanide, alerting the fumigator to dangerous levels of exposure. The record shows no further fatalities after incorporating this improvement, suggesting that carelessness and/or inexperience among workers were major contributing factors to the tragic outcomes. Cyanide fumigations continued through World War II.

Other developments coincided to ease the workload. By agreement at an International Sanitary Convention in 1926, ships from plague-free ports no longer required fumigation unless there was evidence of rats. The Public Health Service hosted teaching conferences on rat-proofing of existing ships and distributed information booklets to shippers to aid them in making appropriate changes. New ship construction now included features that deterred rats from nesting.[77] Changes abroad also helped. US consuls and health officials in Latin America were authorized to make out bills of health as long as the bills complied with instructions. These strategies minimized deportations from San Francisco for health reasons and reduced the number of fumigations.[78]

In 1921 the station chief, Friench Simpson, clearly considered plague the greatest threat to the coast. After ranking the other quarantinable diseases at a lower level, he comments, "There is constantly open the avenue for plague introduction through the escape of plague rats from aboard ship to harborage ashore.... Its control then becomes of great sanitary importance, requiring the cooperation of the entire community and the financing of an expensive sanitary campaign."[79]

The Angel Island Quarantine Station, by the end of the 1920s, had reached its peak size and range of duties. As evidence of success, health conditions were improving in many ports, fewer dead rats were turning up after fumigations, and fewer cases of smallpox burdened the quarantine facilities on Angel Island. By the end of the decade, as the number of arriving vessels with smallpox or other quarantinable disease on board declined, the quarantine barracks remained empty much of the time. In the following years, it made sense to search for simpler quarantine arrangements.

CHAPTER ELEVEN

Final Years

THROUGHOUT THE LATE 1920s and 1930s, fumigations continued, but the number of vessels requiring fumigation declined. Medical officers assigned to ports in foreign countries and in the American possessions—Hawaii, the Philippines, and Puerto Rico—saw to it that more ships arrived with healthy passengers, free of disease. They accomplished this by working in conjunction with consulates and shipping companies. Enhanced small-pox control through vaccination, both in the United States and abroad, was another aid that reduced the need for extensive quarantine facilities. Restrictions on immigration, particularly the Chinese Exclusion Act and the unwritten agreement between Roosevelt and Japan, also lightened the load, as did diminished troop movements. In fact, by the mid-1920s the number of maritime crew inspected at the station who were alien (non-US citizens) well exceeded the number of alien passengers.[1]

To combat rat populations, shipping companies continued to modify old vessels and purchase new ones with rat-proof features. In 1927, in con-junction with new international regulations, the quarantine service began to fumigate only ships with evidence of rats on board, regardless of the port of origin. This saved time and expense and did not result in a resur-gence of infected rats. The practice of scrubbing decks and walls with anti-septics had almost disappeared.

Though smallpox was still prevalent worldwide, it was a less-frequent visitor to San Francisco. There were two instances in 1930, both on American ships. Due to prompt isolation on board the vessels before arrival and the presence of previous immunity in most passengers, only a small number were detained in quarantine.[2] Smallpox prevalence in California was dropping rapidly, too, from more than 3,000 cases in 1930 down to 309 in 1935.[3]

The Great Depression of the 1930s adversely affected shipping volume as it affected everything. In spite of the lean years of the depression, the Golden Gate Bridge and the San Francisco—Oakland Bay Bridge were both constructed over the waters of the Bay, finally linking San Francisco with its neighbors, Marin County in the north and Oakland in the east. By hiking up the hill above Hospital Cove the quarantine station staff could look west and watch the giant towers of the Golden Gate Bridge grow skywards. They would have seen men hanging on to the twin towers, hundreds of feet above water level and often buffeted by high winds. On one occasion an earthquake shook the towers, forcing the workers to cling to the swaying structures. The staff saw the huge cable spinners as they wove 80,000 miles of spliced wire across the enormous bridge span.[4] And, on the day the bridge opened in May 1937, some station employees may have joined the more than 200,000 pedestrians who crossed the bridge, some on foot, others on roller skates, stilts, or unicycles.[5] Looking east, the San Francisco–Oakland Bay Bridge was also visible as construction proceeded. It was really two bridges, meeting on an island midway between the shores. Opening-day celebrations for both bridges, in 1937 and 1936 respectively, were marked by dazzling fireworks, seen easily from Angel Island and temporarily sweeping away thoughts of the ongoing depression.

But the depression was real, and the lower shipping volume in the 1930s translated into fewer disease threats. In 1930–31 466 vessels were fumigated out of a total of 557 inspected, but by 1934 a mere 61 were fumigated out of 448 vessels inspected. By 1935 the count was down to 47 fumigated out of 425 vessels inspected, partly related to waterfront strikes. The International Longshoremen's Association, headed by Henry Bridges, an Australian, closed down the waterfront intermittently starting in May 1934. By July that year the strikes had created more tension and a general strike by all union workers on July 5 paralyzed the city. At the waterfront, national guard troops fired on strikers, a bloody chapter in San Francisco history.

By 1939 only 12 vessels were fumigated out of 500 inspected.[6] As another sign of the lower workload, in October 1930, the chief quarantine officer and the chief of the immigration hospital were combined into one job.[7] San Francisco saw no further cases of plague in rats or humans and no infected rats turned up on incoming ships.

After World War I typhus fever, transmitted by body lice, took advantage of rampant poverty, uprooted homes, and cold weather to infect millions in Europe, especially Eastern Europe. On the American East Coast, where Eastern European immigrants in quest of a new life arrived

in vast numbers, quarantine services used delousing procedures extensively. California, with its limited immigration, had less to fear. In one
instance the station deloused several hundred members of the American
Expeditionary Force who were returning from duty in Siberia. A bathing solution consisting of a mixture of soap and gasoline removed any
lingering lice from their bodies and cyanide gas sterilized their belongings.[8] The station also deloused alien prisoners of war that passed through
during World War II.[9]

Another health problem arose in the winter of 1928–29, an unusual
one: meningitis. Over an eight-month period, on board fourteen ships
from the Philippines and China, a total of 126 steerage passengers came
down with bacterial meningitis.[10] Meningitis is an infection of the fluid
and membranes that surround the brain and spinal cord. The offending
organism in these cases was a *meningococcus*, a bacterium commonly
found in the throat and associated with epidemics. Outbreaks of this
form of meningitis often occur in crowded settings, frequently in military barracks.[11] In this case, the close quarters in steerage class provided the
appropriate setting. Treatment at the time, well before antibiotics, rested
on injecting immune serum into the spinal fluid and providing supportive measures. Such a treatment resulted in prolonged hospital stays.[12]

Since meningitis was not quarantinable, the sick were admitted to
local hospitals, soon overwhelming them. In response, the quarantine
service altered regulations to allow passengers with contagious but non-
quarantinable diseases, and those exposed to them, to receive care at the
station if needed. Healthy passengers underwent a throat culture, and if
found to be harboring the *meningococcus*, were placed with the sick passengers while the remainder spent fourteen days in separate quarters.
In all, more than 2,100 passengers from meningitis-afflicted ships were
held at the station. Fourteen of those came down with meningitis during
their stay.[13] The numbers held in quarantine so overwhelmed the station that President Hoover issued an executive order temporarily halting all passenger traffic from China and the Philippines to San Francisco.
The interruption of passenger arrivals and the onset of spring, with its
moderate weather, allowed the epidemic to finally die out. The following
year, the number of cases mounted again and passengers shipping from
Manila to San Francisco found themselves unable to board unless they
presented evidence of a negative throat culture.[14] The problem eventually disappeared.

In November 1929 an apparently new disease bewildered American doctors. A new, flu-like illness was harassing bird owners. More significant, and alarming, was that the illness often progressed to a more severe, sometimes terminal, stage. Over a six-month period, the illness struck 169 people in sixteen states, 33 of them fatally. Another 16 cases (with 2 deaths) occurred in laboratory workers handling infectious material.[15] The outbreak of the obscure illness coincided with a popular new fad of importing parrots as pets, the majority of them from South America. The birds frequently carried the germ of psittacosis, as the illness was called, and infected those in contact with them. The outbreak was severe enough to induce President Herbert Hoover to impose, by executive order, a ban on importation of parrot-family birds. In a later modification, bird enthusiasts could again import parrots, but only those that first underwent a quarantine period of two weeks before entry.[16]

As the depression ground on and the station's workload lightened, the quarantine buildings on Angel Island remained empty for longer and longer periods. Employees found themselves with less to do as the vacant buildings accumulated dust. The sense of isolation, already a part of island life, grew. As early as 1921, there was consideration of moving the administrative staff to the San Francisco waterfront and doing away with the cooking crew. A waterfront site required land, but diligent searching failed to locate a suitable site. In 1936 the quarantine service raised money and attempted to acquire a three-acre parcel of land on the shore of the Presidio, but the Army balked. Europe was drifting toward war, and when the request reached the secretary of War he commented, "There are no War Department lands in the San Francisco area that can be transferred to the Treasury Department for the purpose desired, without injury to the national defense."[17] Another attempt later met with the same results.[18] Land on Treasure Island, a small, human-made, island about halfway between San Francisco and Oakland, was another possibility, but the Navy occupied this land and, as war approached, used it for pilot training and as an airbase.[19] Searches failed to disclose any other suitable site.

Forced to persevere on Angel Island, the quarantine inspections and immigration inspections of passengers were combined into one function. The lazaret closed and those few passengers found with quarantinable disease were now placed in the San Francisco MHS Hospital; only their contacts were kept at the station for quarantine. The last time the station held passengers in quarantine was in 1935.[20] The quarantine service opened a branch to administer boarding, fumigation, and lookout activities on the second floor of a building at the Fort Mason docks, not far from Meigg's Wharf.[21] When a ship came in, the US Department of Commerce telephoned the arrival of the vessel to this office to initiate the boarding procedure. The Immigration Station, for similar reasons of expense and inconvenience, planned to relocate to the mainland. Construction of a new building in San Francisco began in 1940 to house the immigration hospital, detention quarters, and a number of offices.[22]

That same year saw another change: Pan American clipper ships began flights across the Pacific, a first in commercial aviation. Though the flights were only weekly, a quarantine officer was needed at the San Francisco airport, some miles distant, to conduct incoming and outgoing inspections.[23]

In 1938 more economies were introduced. Ten personnel were dropped from the quarantine station (by not hiring replacements as positions became vacant) and the facility went to a caretaker mode at night. The boarding officers, as in the prior year, remained on the mainland, using a small fumigation office and pier at Fort Mason, though they soon moved to a pier at the foot of Hyde Street.[24]

Change was under way in Washington, too. The Public Health Service moved from the Treasury Department, where it had originated as the MHS, to the newly created Federal Security Agency, though its overall function remained the same. At the FSA it rubbed shoulders with educational and employment bureaus.[25] Correspondence from Angel Island, previously directed to the surgeon general, was now sent to the assistant surgeon general at the foreign quarantine division, reflecting the growing duties of the surgeon general's office and the need to compartmentalize activities.

The noise of war in the 1930s grew ever closer. A more concrete reminder of the conflict materialized when the crew of the German liner *Columbus*, Germany's third-largest passenger liner, arrived at the station. In December 1939, after the *Columbus* had left South America for Germany, it was intercepted about four hundred miles off the coast of Mexico by a British destroyer enforcing a blockade established by England earlier in the war. As the destroyer prepared to capture the ship, the *Columbus*'s captain, Wilhelm Daehne, to avoid letting the liner to fall into British hands, ordered the crew to burn the ship. The crew splashed gasoline throughout the ship, scrambled into lifeboats, and watched while the captain and a few remaining torchmen lit the gasoline. The flames created a fireball within minutes.[26]

The US cruiser *Tuscaloosa,* also tracking *Columbus,* picked up the entire group of 578 drifting crewmembers and transported them to Ellis Island in New York in time for Christmas.[27] Since the United States was not yet at war, the Germans were classified as noncombatants and 512 of the men were transferred to Angel Island to await disposition. The German government paid the tab for their stay.[28]

The station had been idle for some time. Staff levels were reduced and the buildings were looking shabby. Accepting the newcomers was a strain. About two hundred of them found beds at the Immigration Station, which had also reduced its staff, and the remainder occupied the barracks and vacant quarters at Hospital Cove. The Germans generally behaved well and assisted the skeletal staff with various duties. They were allowed fairly frequent shore leave and a couple of sailors even managed to find girlfriends whom they later married.[29] The Red Cross provided them with books, games, and the like.[30]

One night during their stay, angry flames shot out of the Immigration Station's administration building, coloring the sky bright orange. The blaze devoured most of the building, including the famous dining room where the longshoreman and union organizer Harry Bridges had been tried on charges of communism less than a year before. The Germans, roused from their bunks, pitched in to help the firefighters.[31] The fire, apparently originating from faulty wiring, eventually destroyed most of the Immigration Station sleeping quarters and offices and forced the Germans residing there to move to the already crowded quarantine station. This burdened the station's capabilities, though the $1,000-a-day maintenance paid by the German government eased the load on the accounting office. Twenty-three non-German immigrants dislodged by the fire were transferred to a jail for lack of other space and eventually were moved to new quarters on Silver Street in San Francisco.[32] The following year, in view of possible war, the War Department took over the Immigration Station's ten-acre site as a supplement to the Fort McDowell area.[33]

Meanwhile, to house the Germans, a search had located an abandoned Civilian Conservation Corps camp in New Mexico. In part, the move was a response to complaints that some of the crew had been engaging in Nazi propaganda while on leave in San Francisco.[34] Following restoration of the Civilian Conservation Corps camp in the spring, the

Germans moved in. They were unlikely to continue propaganda, as the nearest village was seven miles from the camp and the nearest town a full 75 miles.[35]

Empty again, the quarantine station lapsed back into tranquility. In 1941 only 8 out of 463 vessels received fumigation, and no one was quarantined. Older buildings were torn down and those remaining were fixed up, possibly needlessly. The personnel size fell. The roster listed eighteen employees, but seven worked on the boarding vessel (they still inspected each arriving ship), one was out on illness, and another was filing for disability. Money for quarters and subsistence had been canceled, forcing the men to cook for themselves and find a spot to sleep or go onshore at night. It was truly a skeleton crew.[36] The medical officers now spent most of their time at an office in San Francisco, located in a building at the foot of Hyde Street, which afforded a pleasant view of the Bay and the Golden Gate.[37]

During the prewar period, American merchant shipping believed that it was being threatened by submarine attack. Ships often traveled with naval convoys for protection. Consequently, an entire convoy of up to ninety ships might arrive at a port, needing inspection. This primarily affected ports on the American East Coast; to meet the challenge a 24-hour inspection service was initiated nationally. Defense-related cargoes were particularly at stake.[38] Though the Angel Island personnel participated in the night inspection order, full convoys from the Pacific seldom arrived. Additionally, after America entered the war the foreign quarantine division in Washington was expanded to include members from the Army and the Navy.[39]

The number of immigrants passing through San Francisco fell off considerably. The hospital and residence at the Immigration Station, pending new quarters, moved to a camp in Sharp Park, about fifteen miles from the city. A quarantine service officer traveled to the facility to perform physical examinations and care for the sick.[40]

After the attack on Pearl Harbor, armed forces casualties mounted and were admitted to military hospitals, such as Letterman Hospital in the Presidio. The military considered the quarantine station as a place to manage civilian casualties but by that time the station was minimally staffed and the hospital facilities were no longer in suitable condition. The mattresses, for example, were worn out or on loan to the Immigration Service, and personnel depended on launches to reach the station. Other arrangements were found for injured civilians.[41]

Relations between the station and the Army were a bit strained. The quarantine officials tried multiple times to move the station to the mainland, but the military coveted the desired space. And one day the station chief, Dr. Holdt, found painters, on orders from the Army, camouflaging some of his buildings. The buildings next door at Fort McDowell were not camouflaged, however, nor had the military camouflaged other buildings throughout the Bay Area. Holdt's opinion was that the Army wanted to expand the Fort McDowell hospital by using the quarantine station facilities and that they were using camouflaging as a form of harassment. The Army was unable to provide space on the mainland for a new station as compensation, however, and camouflage painting ceased.[42]

Except for ship inspections and fumigations, the station appears to have seen little activity during the war. Although censorship was in place, neither newspapers nor Public Health Service reports indicate unusual events or action at the station. A number of prisoners of war passed through the island on their way to more permanent camps inland, but they were under the supervision of Fort McDowell officers, and the sick and wounded among them were cared for at Letterman Hospital.[43]

After the great conflict was over, the station remained inactive. The buildings lay empty and dilapidated, casualties of neglect. Only the gentle waves on the small beach at Hospital Cove and winds rustling the trees and grass broke the silence. The Army, downsizing rapidly, lost interest in the adjacent Fort McDowell and moved to close it. The fort's flag was lowered for the final time on August 28, 1946.[44] The only units still functioning on the entire island were the ailing quarantine station and a lighthouse. As a visiting journalist described it, "About 20 officials man the Quarantine Station, confining an occasional inbound seaman or passenger down with disease, according to Dr. W. T. Harrison, regional public health director. The Coast Guard keeps about three men at its lighthouse. Otherwise, the island is deserted."[45]

The quarantine service had been trying to relocate on the mainland since before the war and was frustrated continually by the military's need for space. Those needs evaporated after the war and the Public Health Service sought once again to close the station. In October 1946 the island was declared surplus and turned over to the War Assets Administration, a bureau charged with disposing of no-longer-needed government property. The War Assets Administration ordered an appraisal of its value and a determination of what it might be suited for.[46] Ideas on possible missions for the island flew around like pigeons, ranging from a site for the

United Nations, to park land for Bay Area residents. Even a bridge to the island was proposed, then dropped.[47]

The quarantine station functioned a short time longer, conducting ship inspection and rat-control activities. Sodium fluoroacetate (also called agent 1080), a rat poison that could be left in strategic places as bait to be eaten, began to replace cyanide fumigation. It was safer for personnel, though not for rodents, and avoided time-consuming fumigation. The station finally closed in January 1949. The area remained government property until March 11, 1954, when, as part of a sale to California, the government handed the deed to the thirty-five-acre site at Hospital Cove over to the California governor, Goodwin Knight.[48]

Today Angel Island is a California State Park. California completed acquisition of the entire island in 1963. A small museum on the former quarantine station grounds is the only reminder of the former thirty-five-acre station built to protect the mainland from epidemic disease and to care for victims of those disorders in a compassionate manner. The hectic years the station passed through, working to fend off pestilences that barely exist today, are almost forgotten. The spacious, rough-hewn barracks with assembly-line showers; the huge steam sterilizers through which passed tons of clothing and personal belongings; the giant cauldrons boiling vast amounts of rice, and the lazaretto housing smallpox victims all remain only in memory.

Epilogue

THE ANGEL ISLAND QUARANTINE STATION enjoyed a life span of fifty-eight years, from the opening in 1891 to the closure in 1949. Born out of efforts to control yellow fever in New Orleans, the station's functions in California broadened to include vigilance over cholera, plague, small-pox, and occasionally typhus and other contagious diseases. In general, the activities of the station served the residents of San Francisco well. The only major disappointment was the episode of plague, almost certainly carried ashore surreptitiously by a seafaring rodent.

Duties and procedures at the station progressed over the years. Novel disease challenges and advances in medical knowledge demanded adaptation and change. It might be said that the application of new knowledge is what eventually doomed the quarantine station. As the nature of conta-gious diseases and their modes of transmission were clarified, vaccination rates rose, water supplies improved, and rat control measures gained effi-ciency. Worries about cholera epidemics dwindled, fewer passengers devel-oped smallpox, and plague faded from newspaper headlines. Eventually, the extensive quarantine facilities on Angel Island, which were capable of handling hundreds of people at a time, outlived their usefulness and were abandoned.

The station chiefs of the MHS, later the Public Health Service, after passing rigorous examinations, were assigned in military fashion to the station. They worked long hours in isolated environments and engaged in such diverse activities as inspecting and disinfecting arriving vessels, overseeing hundreds of passengers at a time held in quarantine, treating the ill, and supervising the staff. Meager budgets often hampered their work, and the press and politicians could be unfriendly. The work of the quarantine officers seldom elicited awe or wonder in the way a daring surgeon pioneering a new operation might. Yet the health of an entire community was at stake.

Several men who served on Angel Island achieved admirable careers. Milton Rosenau, after leaving Angel Island, was appointed to head the Hygienic Laboratory of the Public Health Service, Joseph Kinyoun's old workplace. Rosenau then moved to Harvard University as professor of epidemiology and wrote an important textbook, *Preventive Medicine and Hygiene*. In 1936 the University of North Carolina called on him to establish a Division of Public Health in the School of Medicine, an entity that grew into a separate school, with Rosenau as dean.[1]

Rupert Blue, first assigned to Angel Island in 1896 to assist Rosenau in boarding ships, returned twice to San Francisco to carry out plague suppression. After various further assignments, he rose to the office of surgeon general in 1912, the year that the US Public Health and Marine Hospital Service (PHMHS) became the Public Health Service. He served until 1920, shepherding MHS through the trials of World War I and the 1918 influenza epidemic. After 1920 he stepped down and was assigned, as assistant surgeon general, to represent the United States at the Office International d'Hygiène Publique (a forerunner of the World Health Organization), and later at the League of Nations.[2]

Hugh Cumming, after two Angel Island assignments, served in Yokohama and at the Hygienic Laboratory in Washington. He succeeded Rupert Blue as surgeon general in 1920 and occupied that office until 1936. His tenure oversaw the establishment of the National Leprosarium of the United States in Carville, Louisiana; the improvement of medical inspection of immigrants abroad; the creation of a Division of Narcotics (later renamed Division of Mental Hygiene); and the transformation of the Hygienic Laboratory into the National Institutes of Health. Unfortunately, also under his watch, the Public Health Service began the infamous Tuskegee Syphilis Experiment (1932) and did not terminate it until 1972.[3] After retirement from the surgeon general's office, Cumming served as director of the Pan American Sanitary Bureau until 1947.[4]

William Hobdy, who carried out the rat quarantine after the San Francisco earthquake, went on his next assignment to Honolulu. He worked there with the PHMHS for a short time and then opened a private practice. He acted as private physician to Queen Liliuokalani, the last monarch of Hawaii. In 1920 he returned to San Francisco, where he resumed private practice, remaining until his death in 1938.[5]

Joseph Kinyoun did not go to Detroit after his antiplague activity as assigned. Instead, he traveled to Asia to work on plague; while in the Philippines he discovered the parasite causing an important disease of horses.[6] He resigned from the MHS (by that time it was the PHMHS), joined a large pharmaceutical firm, and later was appointed director of the Bacteriology Laboratory of the Washington, DC, Health Department. There he developed an improved smallpox vaccination technique and an improved stain to detect tuberculosis bacilli under the microscope that is still in use today. In World War I he served as an epidemiologist in the United States, investigating typhoid epidemics. Despite requests to write about his experiences he never publicly disclosed details of unethical or illegal behavior toward him in California, including attempts at bribery. He never returned to the modest laboratory where he had started his career. Today, however, a portrait of Kinyoun hangs in the National Institutes of Health to remind visitors of the first director of the fledgling Hygienic Laboratory on Staten Island, the forerunner of that institution.[7]

Walter Wyman ran the MHS until his death in 1911. He also helped found the Pan American Sanitary Bureau, opened in 1902, and served as its director until 1911. He was president of the first two Inter-American Sanitary Conferences and was president of the American Public Health Association in 1902. His involvement in these activities helped create an international sanitary agreement for the control of major epidemic diseases in the western hemisphere. He was an active member of numerous other organizations, particularly those involved with international health. He authorized a survey of leprosy and visited Hawaii to help select a site for a leprosy hospital there.

Under Wyman's stewardship, the MHS expanded to the PHMHS in 1902. He moved the Hygienic Laboratory from Staten Island to Washington, DC, where it undertook studies of a number of infectious diseases. With the passage of the Biologics Control Act in 1902, the laboratory assumed responsibility for the quality of vaccines and other biologics. Eventually it expanded into the National Institutes of Health. Wyman initiated the bulletin, *Public Health Reports,* a publication that compiled health statistics collected at the state level and reported on new developments in public health. He died in 1911, just before the final transition, in 1912, of the PHMHS to the Public Health Service that we know today.[8]

Closing the quarantine station on Angel Island was not a move to abandon quarantine. It reflected changing times. The long ocean voyages that brought so many passengers to American shores were gradually replaced by faster and more comfortable air travel. International air traffic began in the late 1930s, and officers from the San Francisco Quarantine Station made runs to the San Francisco Airport to meet the planes. At first, inspections at the airport were an inconvenient duty added on to regular work. But in the postwar period, air traffic increased exponentially and eventually a separate quarantine office opened for duty at the airport.

The list of diseases subject to quarantine also underwent change and will undoubtedly be altered again as needs dictate. Currently, the list includes, in addition to the five diseases already enumerated, diphtheria, viral hemorrhagic fevers, epidemic-prone strains of influenza, and severe acute respiratory syndromes (severe acute respiratory syndrome [SARS] and Covid-19). Further additions can be made by executive order of the president.[9]

The Division of Global Migration and Quarantine within the Centers for Disease Control and Prevention is currently responsible for quarantine and border inspection activities. The volume of passengers arriving by air far outweighs that arriving by sea in San Francisco, and it is logical that the division office is at the San Francisco Airport. Seagoing passengers today usually step off cruise ships rather than passenger or cargo liners.

Although the threat of plague, cholera, and other diseases that formerly kept health officials in a state of anxiety has almost disappeared, and smallpox has completely disappeared, new hazards have emerged and almost certainly will continue to pose challenges. A dramatic event in recent years was the epidemic of SARS that swept through multiple countries in early 2003, affecting more than eight thousand people worldwide. Jet air travel, a feature of modern times, was important in the disease's rapid spread. More recently, Ebola virus ravaged parts of Africa and, once again, traveled to the United States by air. Because it is transmitted through blood and body fluids, a worldwide epidemic is unlikely.

In 2020 the global epidemic of the Covid-19 virus, a cousin of the SARS virus, has dwarfed other recent epidemics in sheer numbers infected. As fatalities rise, it threatens to rival the 1918 influenza epidemic in severity. Quarantine of the type practiced on Angel Island would be useless with Covid-19 virus. Screening travelers at airports can provide some protection. But, since people are often infected but show no symptoms and the virus is easily transmitted, control at borders is incomplete. Furthermore, individuals are no longer quarantined on an island, but in their homes, in hotels, or in other facilities. As of this writing, vaccination promises to be the most promising method of terminating the epidemic.

The days are over when people toughed it out in rustic and poorly heated quarters on Angel Island, putting up with fires, rainstorms, and isolation as they herded humble steerage passengers into rough barracks for a quarantine. But the story of the San Francisco Quarantine Station is an important one. It is fitting that there remains a small museum at Hospital Cove to remind visitors of the station's important activities, activities from an era when maladies like smallpox and plague circulated in our midst and quarantine procedures were finding their way from early and sometimes misguided stages to a mature state. The museum is also a sober reminder of one small step in the arduous passage of thousands of immigrants to San Francisco, immigrants whose work and whose descendants have made the city one of the most dynamic in the nation.

Acknowledgments

My PROFOUND GRATITUDE goes to the staff of the National Archives and Records Administration, both in San Bruno, California, and in College Park, Maryland. Their promptness and efficiency in providing numerous documents were of inestimable help. Likewise, the staff of the research department of the San Francisco Public Library furnished me with important information and guidance, for which I am grateful, and the library's newspaper files were invaluable. The services and collections at the libraries of the University of California, both in San Francisco and Berkeley, provided essential background material. Additionally, I owe thanks to several local libraries that provided me with volumes that contributed information for this book: A particular appreciation is due to Gina Bardi and Bert Ho at the Maritime Research Center, a centerpiece of the San Francisco Maritime National Historical Park. Here, the attentive staff provided me with the original logbooks of the first days of the station. Stephen Greenberg and John Rees at the National Library of Medicine thankfully provided me with guidance and information. The staff at the Angel Island Conservancy was helpful in locating photographs to enhance the work. I am indebted to the California State Library in Sacramento for their online newspaper files and the California History Room at the California State Library, where Sara Cordes kindly supplied me with photographic material. And a thanks to Phaedra Nations at the Cultural Resources Division, California State Parks Statewide Museum Collections Center, for information and photographs.

I owe much to the staff at the University of Nevada Press. Margaret Dalrymple, who first encouraged me to develop the manuscript into its present form, receives my special thanks. Virginia Fontana, Caddie Dufurrena, and Alison Hope were of great help in editing and shaping the final product.

The availability of online sources of information has reached an astounding level. I particularly appreciate the presence of the Internet

Archive and the Hathi Trust as ready sources of many papers and books that in earlier days would have entailed valuable extra research time.

Last, but not least, I am indebted to the friends and colleagues that took valuable time to review the manuscript and make suggestions. Their ideas and criticisms have helped to improve the manuscript immensely. And I am deeply grateful to my wife, who was a constant source of inspiration and, exercising superhuman patience and understanding, was my most astute critic.

Notes

anon.   anonymous
AR of CGI   *Annual Report of the Commissioner General of Immigration*
AR of NBH   *Annual Report of the National Board of Health*
AR of SFDH   *Annual Report of the San Francisco Department of Health*
AR of SG   *Annual Report of the Surgeon General*
AR of SSG   *Annual Report of the Supervising Surgeon General*
CSBH   California State Board of Health
FQD   foreign quarantine division
grp.   group
JAMA   *Journal of the American Medical Association*
MHS   Marine Hospital Service
MOJMHS   Medical Officer's Journal, US Marine Hospital Service
NARA   National Archives and Records Administration
NBH   National Board of Health
NS   new series
O&O   Occidental and Oriental Steamship Company
PHMHS   Public Health and Marine Hospital Service
PMSS   Pacific Mail Steamship Company
RG   record group
SFChron.   *San Francisco Chronicle*
SFDH   *San Francisco Department of Health*
SFEx.   *San Francisco Examiner*
SFMo.   *San Francisco Morning Call*
SFMR   *San Francisco Municipal Reports*

CHAPTER I. DEATH IN THE HOLD

1. Chinese Exclusion Act of 1882, https://www.ourdocuments.gov/doc.php?doc=47

2. Lucy E. Salyer, *Laws Harsh as Tigers* (Chapel Hill: Univ. of North Carolina Press, 1995), 1–22; Stuart Creighton Miller, *The Unwelcome Immigrant: The American Image of the Chinese, 1785–1882* (Berkeley: Univ. of California Press, 1969), 145–204; Chinese Exclusion Act of 1882, https://www.ourdocuments.gov/doc.php?flash=false&doc=47&page=transcript

3. Erika Lee, *At America's Gates: Chinese Immigration During the Exclusion Era, 1882–1943* (Chapel Hill: Univ. of North Carolina Press, 2005), 25–26.

4. *SFChron.*, February 28, 1882.

5. Salyer, *Laws Harsh as Tigers,* chap. 1.

6. Jonathan Spence, *The Search for Modern China* (New York: W.W. Norton, 1990), 165–88.

7. *SFChron.*, February 28, 1882.

8. Lee, *At America's Gates,* 43–44.

9. The Passenger Act of 1882 "An act to regulate the carriage of passengers by sea," in *Statutes at Large of the United States of America,* vol. 22 (1881–83) (Wash., DC: GPO, 1883), 186–91, 186–91, https://tile.loc.gov/storage-services/service/ll/llsl//llsl-c47/llsl-c47.pdf. The history of steerage conditions is discussed in Robert E. Barde, *Immigration at the Golden Gate: Passenger Ships, Exclusion, and Angel Island* (Westport, CT: Praeger, 2008), 82–142.

10. "Health Officer's Report," *SFMR 1882* (San Francisco: Board of Supervisors, 1882), 361–62.

11. *AR of NBH,* Appx. N (Wash., DC: GPO, 1882), 577.

12. Almost the entire story of the *Altonower* is told in *SFChron.*, May 7, 1882, through June 1882, and in *SFMo.*, May 7, 1882, through June 1882. A few supplementary notes are added below.

13. "Health Officer's Report," *SFMR 1877,* 394–99; "Health Officer's Report," *SFMR 1873,* 336–37.

14. Joan B. Trauner, "The Chinese as Medical Scapegoats in San Francisco, 1870–1905," *California History* 57, no. 1 (1978), 70–87.

15. "Health Officer's Report," *SFMR 1881,* 254–55.

16. "Health Officer's Report" 1881, 315.

17. *SFChron.*, February 14, 1882.

18. *SFChron.*, May 7, 1882, through June 1882; *SFMo.*, May 7, 1882, through June 1882.

19. *New York Herald,* May 25, 1882.

20. *AR of NBH 1882,* Appx. N, 573–78.

21. *AR of NBH 1882,* Appx. N, 576–77.

22. *New York Herald,* May 25, 1882; *SFChron.*, May 7, 1882 through June 1882; *SFMo.*, May 7, 1882 through June 1882.

23. *SFMo.*, May 27, 1892; *SFChron.*, May 27, 1892.

24. *SFMo.*, May 28, 1892.

25. *AR of NBH 1882,* Appx. N, 571–72.

26. *AR of NBH 1882,* 33–34.

CHAPTER 2. THE ORIGINS OF QUARANTINE IN AMERICA

1. For discussion of this topic see Charles-Edward Amory Winslow, *The Conquest of Epidemic Disease: A Chapter in the History of Ideas* (Princeton, NJ: Princeton Univ. Press, 1943), chap. 1–8; and L. Fabian Hirst, *The Conquest of Plague: A Study of the Evolution of Epidemiology* (Oxford: Oxford Univ. Press, 1953), chap. 1–3.

2. Philip Ziegler, *The Black Death* (New York: John Day Co, 1969).

3. Hirst, *Conquest of Plague,* 152–87. An entire issue of the *Journal of Hygiene* is devoted to this topic: vol. 6, no. 4 (1906): 422–526.

4. Mark Harrison, *Contagion: How Commerce Has Spread Disease* (New Haven, CT: Yale Univ. Press, 2012), 11–13; Ralph C. Williams, *The US Public Health Service, 1798–1950* (Wash., DC: Commissioned Officers Association of the Public Health Service, 1951), 64–65.

5. Paul S. Sehdev, "The Origin of Quarantine," *Clinical Infectious Diseases* 35, no. 9 (2002): 1071–72; Josip Matovinovic, "A Short History of Quarantine," *University of*

Michigan Medical Center Journal 35, no. 4 (1969): 224–28; Susan Mosher Stuard, *A State of Deference: Ragusa/Dubrovnik in the Medieval Centuries* (Philadelphia: Univ. of Pennsylvania Press, 1992), 44–48.

6. Maria C. Valsecchi, "Mass Plague Graves Found on Venice 'Quarantine' Island," *National Geographic News*, Aug. 29, 2007, http://news.nationalgeographic.com/news/2007/08/070829-venice-plague.html

7. John Howard, *An Account of the Principle Lazzarettos in Europe, with Various Papers Relative to the Plague; Together with Further Observations on Some Foreign Prisons and Hospitals; and Additional Remarks on the Present State of Those Great Britain and Ireland* (London: William Eyres, 1789), 3–23.

8. John Macauley Eager, "The Early History of Quarantine: Origin of Sanitary Measures Directed Against Yellow Fever," *Yellow Fever Institute Bulletin #12* (Wash., DC: US Department of the Treasury, PHMHS, 1903), 19–23.

9. Gian Franco Gensini, Magdi H. Yacoub, and Andrea A. Conti, "The Concept of Quarantine in History: From Plague to SARS," *Journal of Infection* 49, no. 4 (2004): 257–61.

10. Harrison, *Contagion*, 40–41, 180; Alexander Chase-Levenson, "Early Nineteenth-Century Mediterranean Quarantine as a European System," in *Quarantine: Local and Global Histories*, ed. Alison Bashford (New York: Palgrave MacMillan, 2016), 40.

11. Chase-Levenson, "Early Nineteenth-Century Mediterranean Quarantine as a European System," 43–44.

12. G. M. Findlay, "The First Recognized Epidemic of Yellow Fever," *Transactions of the Royal Society of Tropical Medicine* 35, no. 3 (1941): 143–54; Henry Rose Carter, *Yellow Fever: An Epidemiological and Historical Study of Its Place of Origin* (Baltimore: Williams & Wilkins, 1931), 81–85.

13. Findlay, "First Recognized Epidemic"; Carter, *Yellow Fever*.

14. Harrison, *Contagion*, 21–22.

15. R. Pollitzer, *Cholera* (Geneva: World Health Organization, 1959), 11–50; Dhiman Barua, "History of Cholera," in *Cholera*, ed. Dhiman Barua and William B Greenough III (New York: Springer, 1992), 1–7; Fielding H. Garrison, *An Introduction to the History of Medicine* (Philadelphia: W. B. Saunders, 1929), 269–71.

16. Richard L. Guerrant, David H. Walker, and Peter F. Weller, *Tropical Infectious Disease: Principles, Pathogens, and Practice* (Philadelphia: Churchill Livingstone—Elsevier, 2006), 273–80.

17. Peter Baldwin, *Contagion and the State in Europe* (Cambridge: Cambridge Univ. Press, 1999), 41–45; Barua, "History of Cholera," 8–11.

18. Charles E. Rosenberg, *The Cholera Years* (Chicago: Univ. of Chicago Press, 1962), 13–39.

19. Rosenberg, *Cholera Years*, 48.

20. Rosenberg, *Cholera Years*, 115; J. S. Chalmers, *The Conquest of Cholera* (New York: Macmillan, 1938), 239–42.

21. Barua, "History of Cholera," 14.

22. Norman Howard-Jones, *The Scientific Background of the International Sanitary Conferences, 1851–1938* (Geneva: World Health Organization, 1975), 12–16.

23. Howard-Jones, *The Scientific Background of the International Sanitary Conferences*, 46–57.

24. Frank Fenner, Donald A. Henderson, Isao Arita, Zdenek Jezek, and Ivan D. Ladnyi, *Smallpox and Its Eradication* (Geneva: World Health Organization, 1988), 1–55.

25. George M. Sternberg, *Report on the Etiology and Prevention of Yellow Fever* (Wash., DC: GPO, 1890), 43–49.

26. Alfred Perry, "Report of Sanitary Inspector, Fourth District," *Annual Report of the Board of Health to the General Assembly of Louisiana, December 31st, 1872* (New Orleans: Board of Health, 1873), 92–99; Alfred Perry, "Report of Sanitary Inspector, Fourth District," *Annual Report of the Board of Health to the General Assembly of Louisiana, December 31st, 1873* (New Orleans: Board of Health, 1874), 188–93.

27. Alfred Perry, "Effectual External Sanitary Regulations without Delay to Commerce," *Public Health Reports and Papers Presented at the Meetings of the American Public Health Association in the Year 1873* (New York: Hurd and Houghton, 1873), 437–40. The paper was republished in slightly modified form as Alfred W. Perry, "Quarantine without Obstruction to Commerce," *New Orleans Medical and Surgical Journal,* N. S. 1 (1874): 567–72.

28. Perry, "Effectual External Sanitary Regulations," 437.

29. Joseph Lister, "Illustrations of the Antiseptic System of Treatment in Surgery," *The Lancet* Nov. 30 (1867): 668–69.

30. Robert Koch,"Die Aetiologie der Milzbrand-Krankheit, Begründet auf die Entwicklungsgeschichte des Bacillus Anthracis," *Beiträge zur Biologie der Pflanzen* 2, no. 2 (1876): 277–310.

31. Williams, *US Public Health Service,* 72.

32. Jo Ann Carrigan, *The Saffron Scourge: A History of Yellow Fever in Louisiana, 1796–1905,* (Lafayette: Center for Louisiana Studies, 1994), 406–7.

33. *Biennial Report of the Louisiana State Board of Health 1883–84* (Baton Rouge: Louisiana State Board of Health, 1884), 161.

34. Carrigan, *Saffron Scourge,* 114–15; Margaret Humphreys, *Yellow Fever and the South* (Baltimore: Johns Hopkins Univ. Press, 1992), 60–61.

35. Ellis, *Yellow Fever and Public Health,* 61–67.

36. See, e.g., *New Orleans Daily Picayune,* May 6, 1884; and *Albuquerque Morning Democrat,* Jun. 12, 1887.

37. Editorial, *The Sanitarian* 9, no. 95 (1881): 86–88.

38. Humphreys, *Yellow Fever,* 98–99; Ellis, *Yellow Fever,* 100–102; Obituary, *The Times-Picayune,* August 24, 1922.

39. Editorial, *The Sanitarian* 13, no. 176 (1884): 69 (quote).

40. Joseph Holt, "Address to the Louisiana State Board of Health," *New Orleans Medical and Surgical Journal,* 11 (May) (1884): 890–96.

41. Carrigan, *Saffron Scourge,* 135–37.

42. Joseph Holt, "The Quarantine System of Louisiana—Methods of Disinfection Practiced," *Public Health Papers and Reports Presented at the Meetings of the American Public Health Association* 13 (1887): 161–87.

43. Joseph Holt, *The New Quarantine System,* reprint from *New Orleans Medical and Surgical Journal* (New Orleans, LA: New Orleans Medical Publishing Association, 1885).

44. John B. Hamilton, "Quarantine Near New Orleans," *Weekly Abstract of Sanitary Reports* 3, no. 26 (1888): 117–47; first quote on 117, second quote on 138.

45. Lucien F. Salomon, "The Louisiana Quarantine System and Its Contemplated Improvement," *Public Health Papers and Reports Presented at the Meetings of the American Public Health Association* 14 (1888): 110–15.

46. John H. Rauch, *Report of an Inspection of the Atlantic and Gulf Quarantines between the St. Lawrence and Rio Grande* (Springfield: Illinois State Board of Health, 1886), 26–29.

47. H. B. Horlbeck, "Maritime Sanitation at Ports of Arrival," *Public Health Papers and Reports Presented at the Meetings of the American Public Health Association* 16 (1890): 116–23.

48. *Tenth Biennial Report of the State Board of Health of California for the Fiscal Years from June 30, 1886 to June 30, 1888* (Sacramento: State Printing Office, 1888), 252–55; quote on 255.

49. John B. Hamilton, "Report on the Sanitation of Ships and Quarantine," *AR of SSG of MHS 1890* (Wash., DC: GPO), 93.

50. Anon., "Louisiana Quarantine," *JAMA* 21, no. 18 (1893): 662–63.

51. The complicated issues are nicely summarized in John Duffy, *The Sanitarians* (Chicago: Univ. of Chicago Press, 1990), 162–72; and Humphreys, *Yellow Fever*, 13–14.

52. Excellent accounts of the history of the MHS and its evolution into the Public Health Service can be found in Williams, *US Public Health Service*; and Bess Furman in consultation with Ralph C. Williams, *A Profile of the US Public Health Service, 1798–1950* (Wash., DC: GPO, 1973).

53. Humphreys, *Yellow Fever*, 45–111.

54. Williams, *US Public Health Service*, 28–32.

55. Fitzhugh Mullan, *Plagues and Politics: The Story of the US Public Health Service* (New York: Basic Books, 1989), 19–22; Furman, *A Profile of the US Public Health Service*, 121–49.

56. Williams, *The US Public Health Service*, 472–75; William B. Atkinson, ed., *The Physicians and Surgeons of the United States* (Philadelphia: Charles Robson, 1878), 154–55; *American National Biography* (New York: Oxford Univ. Press, 1999), 836–37.

57. Furman, *A Profile of the US Public Health Service*, 121–49.

58. John M. Woodworth, "The General Subject of Quarantine with Special Reference to Cholera and Yellow Fever," in *Transactions of the International Medical Congress of Philadelphia of 1876*, ed. John Ashhurst (Philadelphia: International Medical Congress, 1877), 1059.

59. Furman, *A Profile of the US Public Health Service*, 136–39; J. M. Michael, "The National Board of Health: 1879–1883," *Public Health Reports* 126, no. 1 (2011): 123–29.

60. Humphreys, *Yellow Fever*, 62–65; John Duffy, ed., *The Rudolph Matas History of Medicine in Louisiana* (Baton Rouge: Louisiana State Univ. Press, 1915), vol. 2, 469–78; *AR of SSG of the MHS 1888*, 12–21.

61. Williams, *The US Public Health Service*, 475–77; Furman, *A Profile of the US Public Health Service*, chap. 6; Michael, "National Board of Health," 123–29.

62. Humphreys, Yellow Fever, 128–29.

63. *AR of SSG 1888*, 12–17.

64. Michael, "The National Board of Health," 123–29.

65. Williams, *The US Public Health Service*, 476.

66. Victoria Harden, *Inventing the NIH: Federal Biomedical Research Policy, 1887–1937* (Baltimore: Johns Hopkins Univ. Press, 1986).

67. "U.S. Public Health Service Commissioned Corps: History," https://web.archive .org/web/20121020040704/http://www.usphs.gov/aboutus/history.aspx; C. E. Coop and

H. M. Ginzburg, "The Revitalization of the Public Health Service Commissioned Corps," *Public Health Reports* 104, no. 2 (1989): 105–10.

68. Hobdy to John W. Colbert, Aug. 22, 1906, NARA San Bruno, RG 90, box 3, vol. 30, 50–51.

69. *AR of SSG 1888*, 11.

CHAPTER 3. CHOOSING A SITE

1. F. William Blaisdell and Moses Grossman, *Catastrophes, Epidemics, and Neglected Diseases: San Francisco General Hospital and the Evolution of Public Care* (San Francisco: San Francisco General Hospital Foundation, 1999), 152–54; Chalmers, *Conquest of Cholera*, 193–259; Henry Harris, California's Medical Story (San Francisco: J. W. Stacey, 1932), 79–80.

2. *California State Assembly Statutes: The Statutes of California Passed at the First Session of the Legislature* (San Jose: State of California, 1850), 162–70.

3. "Amendment to Health Report," *SFMR 1866* (San Francisco: Board of Supervisors, 1866), 413–14.

4. "Board of Health," *SFMR 1865*, 394–95; "Health Officer's Report," *SFMR 1866*, 222–24.

5. "Amendment to Municipal Reports: Health Department," *SFMR 1866*, 413–14.

6. George Rosen, *A History of Public Health: Expanded Edition* (Baltimore: Johns Hopkins Univ. Press, 1993), 209–26.

7. Henry Gibbon, "The Variolous Epidemic in San Francisco in 1868," *Transactions of the American Medical Association* 20 (1869): 528–42.

8. George D. Lyman, "The Beginnings of California's Medical History," *California and Western Medicine* 23, no. 5 (1925): 561–76; quote on 570.

9. Alonzo Phelps, *Contemporary Biography of California's Representative Men* (San Francisco: A. L. Bancroft, 1881), 82–84.

10. Guy P. Jones, "Thomas Logan, MD, Organizer of California State Board of Health and a Co-founder of the California Medical Association," *California and Western Medicine* 63, no. 1 (1945): 6–10.

11. Harris, *California's Medical Story*, 164–65.

12. *Biennial Report, State Board of Health of California 1870–1* (Sacramento: State of California, 1871), 22; *An Act to Establish a Quarantine for the Bay and Harbor of San Francisco, and Sanitary Laws for the City and County of San Francisco* (Sacramento: State of California, 1870).

13. *An Act to Establish a Quarantine*, 6.

14. *An Act to Establish a Quarantine*, 8.

15. Anon., "The Quarantine Station at San Francisco," *Occidental Medical Times* 3, no. 1 (1889): 34.

16. "Health Officer's Report," *SFMR 1873*, 336–37.

17. "Report of Quarantine Officer," *AR of SFDH 1877* (San Francisco: SFDH, 1877), 50–53. "Report of Health Officer," *AR of SFDH 1877*, 10.

18. "Report of Quarantine Officer," *AR of SFDH 1877*, 52–53.

19. Quoted in Trauner, "The Chinese as Medical Scapegoats," 70–87.

20. Anon., "Quarantine at New York," *Harper's Weekly* 23, no. 1184 (Sept. 6) (1879): 706.

21. "Health Officer's Report," *SFMR 1879*, 180–81; quote on 181.

22. John Soennichsen, *Miwoks to Missiles: A History of Angel Island* (Tiburon, CA: Angel Island Association, 2005), 5–74.

23. "Report of the Committee on State Quarantine," *Appendix to the Journals of the Senate and Assembly of the 26th Session of the Legislature of the State of California*, vol. 3 (Sacramento: State Printing Office, 1885), 17–19.

24. Soennichsen, *Miwoks to Missiles*, 83–84.

25. *Eighth Biennial Report, State Board of Health of California 1882–84*, 17–19.

26. *AR of NBH 1882*, 33–34, Appx. N, 573–78; quote on 573; Soennichsen, *Miwoks to Missiles*, 83–84.

27. *AR of NBH 1882*, and Appx. N, 573–74.

28. *Ninth Biennial Report, State Board of Health of California 1884–6*, 13.

29. Editorial, *Pacific Medical Journal* 25, no. 1 (1883): 381–82.

30. "A History of UCSF: People: R. Beverly Cole (1829–1901," http://history.library.ucsf.edu/cole.html

31. *Ninth Biennial Report CSBH*, 13–15.

32. *Ninth Biennial Report CSBH*, 16–23.

33. *Ninth Biennial Report CSBH*, 22.

34. *Ninth Biennial Report CSBH*, 23–24.

35. *SFChron.*, May 31, 1888. (The result of the negotiations was the Scott Act, passed unilaterally by the US Congress.); "An Act to Prohibit the Coming of Chinese Laborers to the United States," 1888, 50th Congress, Sess. I, chap. 1015, 476, https://college.cengage.com/history/ayers_primary_sources/prohibitcoming_chinese_laborers.htm

36. "Quarantine Officer's Report," *SFMR 1888*, 526.

37. *SFChron.*, May 24, May 27, 1887.

38. "Health Officer's Report," *SFMR 1888*, 465–72.

39. *Tenth Biennial Report, CSBH 1886–8*, 136–41; "Health Officer's Report," *SFMR 1888*, 465–72.

40. "Health Officer's Report," *SFMR FY 1888*, 468; *SFMo.*, Jan. 22, 1888.

41. *SFChron.*, Jan. 23, 1888.

42. *Pacific Medical and Surgical Journal 31*, no. 3 (1888): S. S. Herrick, "Review of Smallpox in San Francisco from May 3, 1887 to March 21, 1888," *Pacific Medical and Surgical Journal 31*, no. 4 (1888): 207–13; *Tenth Biennial Report CSBH 1886–8*, 43.

43. "Health Officer's Report," *SFMR 1888*, 471.

44. "Quarantine Officer's Report," *SFDH 1888*, 64.

45. Ibid., 64.

46. Editorial, *Pacific Medical and Surgical Journal* 31, no. 6 (1888): 347–49.

47. *AR of SFDH 1888*, 10; *Daily Alta California*, Mar. 7, 1888.

48. Editorial, *Pacific Medical and Surgical Journal* 31, no. 8 (1888): 474.

49. Editorial, *Pacific Medical and Surgical Journal* 31, no. 8 (1888): 474; *SFChron.*, Jul. 24, 1888.

50. *SFChron.*, Nov. 12, 1888.

51. *SFChron.*, Mar. 13, 1889.

52. *SFChron.*, Mar. 13, 1889; Soennichsen, *Miwoks to Missiles*, 84.

53. *SFChron.*, Dec. 18, 1889.

54. *SFChron.*, Mar. 15, 1890.

55. *Tenth Biennial Report CSBH* 1886–88, 42–44.

56. Surgeon General to Station, Sept. 1, 1893, NARA San Bruno, RG 90, box 13, vol. 2.

57. In January 1889 Congress established rankings for the MHS officers. The lowest rank was assistant surgeon, the next highest was passed assistant surgeon, and the highest rank was surgeon. Promotions were conditional on passing an examination at each level. Officers were appointed by the president with consent of the Senate. Wyman's title as chief was supervising surgeon general, which was changed to surgeon general in 1902. (See "An act to regulate appointments in the Marine Hospital Service of the United States," 50th Congress, Sess. 2, 1889.)

58. *SFChron.*, Oct. 19, 1890, Dec. 7, 1890, Jan. 29, 1891; *SFMo.*, Jan. 29, 1891; *AR of SSG 1892,* 73–85.

CHAPTER 4. GROWING PAINS

1. *SFChron.*, Apr. 26 and 27, 1891.

2. The San Francisco MHS Hospital, opened in 1875, was located at the Presidio, the principal military base in the area. The MHS operated it for the care of seamen.

3. *SFMo.*, Apr. 27, 1891.

4. William Issel and Robert W. Cherney, *San Francisco, 1865–1932: Politics, Power, and Urban Development* (Berkeley: Univ. of California Press, 1986), 58–63.

5. There are many histories that have been written of San Francisco. Among them are Oscar Lewis, *San Francisco: Mission to Metropolis* (Berkeley: Howell-North Books, 1966); William Bullough, *The Blind Boss & His City: Christopher Augustine Buckley and Nineteenth-Century San Francisco* (Berkeley: Univ. of California Press, 1979); John B. McGloin, *San Francisco: The Story of a City* (San Rafael: Presidio Press, 1978); Doris Muscatine, *Old San Francisco: The Biography of a City from Early Days to the Earthquake* (New York: G.P. Putnam's Sons, 1975); Issel and Cherney, *San Francisco, 1865–1932*; and Gray Brechin, *Imperial San Francisco: Urban Power, Earthly Ruin* (Berkeley: Univ. of California Press, 1999).

6. Arthur Gold, *The Divine Sarah: A Life of Sarah Bernhardt* (New York: Knopf, 1991).

7. *SFEx.*, Apr. 24, 1891; *SFChron.*, Apr. 27, 1891.

8. *SFChron.*, Apr. 26, 1891.

9. *SFChron.*, Apr. 26, 1891.

10. *SFChron.*, Apr. 26, 1891.

11. *SFMo.*, Apr. 26, 1891.

12. *SFMo.*, Apr. 26, 1891.

13. *SFMo.*, Apr. 26, 1891.

14. Anna Coxe Toogood, *A Civil History of Golden Gate National Recreation Area and Point Reyes National Seashore* (Wash., DC: Historic Preservation Branch, National Park Service, US Department of the Interior, 1980), vol. 1, 326–27. *SFChron.*, Apr. 30, 1891.

15. *AR of SSG of the MHS 1892* (Wash., DC: GPO, 1892), 80.

16. *AR of SSG of the MHS 1892,* 78–79.

17. *SFChron.*, Apr. 30, 1891.

18. *SFChron.*, Apr. 30, 1891.

19. *SFChron.*, Jun 3, 1891.

20. *SFChron.*, Jun. 3, 1891.

21. Toogood, *A Civil History*, vol. 1, 326–27.

22. Toogood, *A Civil History*, vol. 1, 327–28.

23. Williams, *US Public Health Service*, 477–79.

24. "Walter Wyman (1891–1911)," http://wayback.archive-it.org/3929/20171201191736 /https://www.surgeongeneral.gov/about/previous/biowyman.html

25. In 1889 Congress established ranks for MHS officers. The first rank, after passing entry examinations, was assistant surgeon. The next grade, awarded after at least four years of service and passing another examination, was passed assistant surgeon. The final and highest grade was surgeon, reached after another examination.

26. Medical Officer's Journal, US Marine Hospital Service (MOJMHS), Jun. 15 through Sep. 5, 1891. The journal is located at the Maritime Research Center, San Francisco Maritime National Historical Park, San Francisco; *AR of SSG 1892*, 76–85. The author discovered that there is an additional medical officer's journal at the National Library of Medicine covering the years subsequent to the journal cited in this book. Because of the Covid epidemic, it could not be accessed. However, the voluminous correspondence of the medical officers in charge of the station during the entire period was reviewed, and the author believes that little is missing from the narrative.

27. MOJMHS, Jun. 30 through Nov 23, 1891.

28. MOJMHS, Dec. 21, 1892, May 12, 1893; *AR of SSG 1892*, 83.

29. *SFChron.*, Dec. 21, 1891.

30. Don MacGillivray, *Captain Alex MacLean: Jack London's Sea Wolf* (Vancouver, BC: Univ. of British Columbia Press, 2008), 87–94.

31. All events involving *City of Peking* are from MOJMHS, Dec. 20, 1891, to Jan. 9, 1892.

32. *SFChron.*, Jan. 2, 1892.

33. MOJMHS, Jan. 4, 1892.

34. MOJMHS, Jan. 20–Feb. 28, 1892.

35. *SFChron.*, Jan. 28, 1892.

36. *SFChron.*, Jan. 30, 1892.

37. *SFMo.*, Jan. 28, Feb. 2, 1892.

38. MOJMHS, Jan. 20–Feb. 28, 1892.

39. *SFChron.*, Jan. 31, 1892.

40. MOJMHS, Feb. 9–10, 1892.

41. MOJMHS, Mar. 1–30, 1891.

42. *SFChron.*, Apr. 3, 1892.

43. MOJMHS, Apr. 1–5, 1892.

44. MOJMHS, Apr. 16, 1892.

45. MOJMHS, May 2, 1892.

46. MOJMHS, May 5–14, 1892.

47. Surgeon General to Station, May 13, 1892, NARA San Bruno, box 13, vol. 1.

48. O.L. Spaulding, assistant secretary to the Treasury, to Wyman, June 7, 1892, NARA SB, RG 90, Box 13, vol. 1.

49. MOJMHS, May 1892.

50. MOJMHS, May 21, 1892.

51. *AR of SSG 1892*, 84.

52. MOJMHS, Feb. 2, Feb. 5, 1893.

53. *AR of SSG 1892*, 82.

54. MOJMHS, Mar. 1 and 2, 1893.

55. MOJMHS, Mar. 6, 1893.

56. MOJMHS, Apr. 13, 1893

57. MOJMHS, Jan. 11, 1894.

58. *AR of SSG 1894*, 219–20.

59. *AR of SSG 1895*, 297–300.

60. *AR of SSG 1895*, 297–300.

61. *AR of SSG 1896*, 548–49.

62. *AR of SSG 1896*, 546–49.

63. *Bureau Circular No. 191*, Treasury Dept., Nov. 16, 1892.

64. *AR of SSG 1895*, 297.

65. MOJMHS, May 12, 1893.

66. *AR of SSG 1894*, 342.

CHAPTER 5. TWO COMPETING SERVICES

1. "Report of Quarantine Officer," *SFMR 1897–1900; SFChron.*, Aug. 26, 1899.

2. Surgeon General to Station, Jun. 14, 1892, NARA San Bruno RG 90, box 13, vol. 1.

3. *SFMo.*, Mar. 7, 1895.

4. *AR of SSG 1895*, 299–300.

5. *AR of SSG 1895*, 300; *AR of SSG 1896*, 546–53.

6. Furman, *A Profile of the US Public Health Service*, 214.

7. *AR of SSG 1896*, 1024–34.

8. Mark M. Skubik, "Public Health Politics and the San Francisco Plague Epidemic of 1900–1904," Master's Thesis, San Jose State Univ., 2002, 38.

9. *AR of SSG 1896*, 957.

10. *SFChron.*, Jul. 2, 1896.

11. *AR of SSG 1897*, 550.

12. *SFChron.*, Jul. 2, 1896.

13. *SFChron.*, Oct. 11, 1896.

14. *SFEx.*, Jul. 3, 1896.

15. Skubik, "Public Health Politics," 40–41; quote in *SFChron.*, Jul. 3, 1896.

16. *SFChron.*, Jul. 5, 1896.

17. *SFMo.*, Jul. 3, 1896.

18. *SFChron.*, Oct. 11, 1896.

19. *AR of SSG 1897*, 537–58.

20. Anon., "Dr. Hamilton Resigns–Says He Has Been Driven out of Office by Surgeon-General Wyman," *Indiana Medical Journal* 15, no. 5 (1896): 179–80.

21. *AR of SSG 1897*, 537–41.

22. All the correspondence is in *AR of SSG 1897*, 537–58.

23. *AR of SSG 1897*, 543.

24. *AR of SSG 1896,* 959–64 (quote on 963).

25. Quoted in Skubik, "Public Health Politics," 31.

26. *SFChron.,* Apr. 12, 1897.

27. *San Francisco Call,* Jan. 21, 1897.

28. Quote is in *AR of SSG 1897,* 546–47; *United States Quarantine Laws and Regulations, February 24, 1893* (Wash., DC: GPO, 1893), Sec. 3.

29. *SFChron.,* May 19, 1897; *AR of SSG 1897,* 554–55.

30. *SFChron.,* May 19, 1897; quote is in *AR of SSG 1897,* 547.

31. *AR of SSG 1897,* 558.

32. *SFChron.,* Sept. 13, Sept. 14, 1897.

33. *AR of SSG 1897,* 559.

34. *AR of SSG 1900,* 645.

35. Editorial, *Pacific Medical and Surgical Journal* 42, no. 4 (1899): 244.

36. Furman, *A Profile of the US Public Health Service,* 220–21; Anon., "In Honor of Dr. Joseph J. Kinyoun, U.S. Marine Hospital Service," *Georgetown College Journal* 27, no. 9 (1899): 420–22.

37. *Public Health Reports* 14, no. 27 (1899): 1066–67.

38. *SFChron.,* Jun. 28, 1899; *Public Health Reports* 14, no. 33 (1899): 1313–15.

39. *SFChron.,* Jun. 30, 1899.

40. *SFChron.,* Jul. 3, 1899.

41. *SFChron.,* Jul. 3–4, 1899; *AR of SSG 1900,* 646–53.

42. MOJMHS, Jul. 2, 1899.

43. *AR of SSG 1900,* 650.

44. *SFChron.,* Jun. 26 to Aug. 14, 1899; *AR of SSG 1899,* 650.

45. The press frenzy is detailed in Robert Barde, "Prelude to the Plague: Public Health and Politics at America's Pacific Gateway, 1899," *Journal of the History of Medicine* 58, no. 3 (2003): 153–86.

46. *AR of SSG 1900,* 440.

47. *AR of SSG 1900,* 653.

48. *AR of SSG 1900,* 653.

49. *SFChron.,* Aug. 26, 1899.

50. *SFChron.,* Aug. 23, 1899.

51. *SFChron.,* Aug. 25, 1899.

52. *AR of SSG 1900,* 653–55; quote on 655.

53. *Biennial Report of the Board of Health of California 1898–1900,* 11–12.

54. *AR of SSG 1900,* 655.

CHAPTER 6. PLAGUE IN THE CITY

1. Spelling of the name varies. The spelling here is taken from Guenter B. Risse, *Plague, Fear, and Politics in San Francisco's Chinatown* (Baltimore: Johns Hopkins University Press, 2012).

2. W. H. Kellogg, "The Plague: Report of Cases," *Occidental Medical Times* 14, no. 7 (1900): 197–207. Risse states that Wong actually died in a hall of tranquility, which is a room in a coffin shop where Chinese who are near death could expire and be assured a proper burial. *Plague, Fear, and Politics,* 50–51. Although the Marine Hospital Service and

the officer in charge of the Angel Island Station were intimately involved in the early phase of the plague epidemic, the story is somewhat peripheral to the main function of the station as a maritime quarantine service. The account here will, therefore, be brief and is derived in large part from secondary sources. There are excellent accounts of the San Francisco plague epidemic that the reader may consult, such as Risse, *Plague, Fear, and Politics*; Marilyn Chase, *The Barbary Plague: The Black Death in Victorian San Francisco* (New York: Random House, 2003); L. G. Lipson, "Plague in San Francisco: The United States Marine Hospital Service Commission to Study the Existence of Plague in San Francisco," *Annals of Internal Medicine* 77, no. 2 (1972): 303–10; Guenter B. Risse, "Science Contested: Bacteriologists and Bubonic Plague in San Francisco," unpublished lecture, Conference on the Laboratory in 20th Century Medicine: Historical Perspectives, University of California, San Francisco, January 22, 1998, https://www.researchgate.net /publication/301765393_Science_Contested_Bacteriologists_and_Bubonic_Plague_in _San_Francisco; Philip A. Kalisch, "The Black Death in Chinatown: Plague and Politics in San Francisco, 1900–1904," *Arizona and the West* 14, no. 2 (1972): 113–16; Mark M. Skubik, "Public Health Politics and the San Francisco Plague Epidemic of 1900–1904," PhD diss. (San Francisco: San Francisco State University, 2002).

3. "Report of Board of Health: Report of the Bacteriologist," *SFMR 1900*, 538–43.

4. Risse, *Plague, Fear, and Politics*, 82–83.

5. *SFChron.*, Mar. 8, 1900.

6. Risse, *Plague, Fear, and Politics*, 184–87.

7. *SFChron.*, Mar. 14, 1900.

8. *SFChron.*, Mar. 14, 25, 27, 1900.

9. *SFChron.*, Mar. 27, 1900.

10. *SFChron.*, Jun. 3, 1900.

11. *AR of SSG 1900*, 20–21; Wyman to Surgeon Gassaway, MHS Hospital, San Francisco, Mar. 8, 1900, NARA San Bruno, RG 90, box 16, vol. 3.

12. Selman A. Waksman, *The Brilliant and Tragic Life of W. M. W. Haffkine, Bacteriologist* (New Brunswick, NJ: Rutgers Univ. Press, 1964), 45; Barbara Hawgood, "Waldemar Mordecai Haffkine, CIE (1860–1930): Prophylactic Vaccination against Cholera and Bubonic Plague in British India," *Journal of Medical Biography* 15, no. 1 (2007): 9–19.

13. K. F. Meyer, et al., "Plague Immunization. I. Past and Present Trends," *Journal of Infectious Diseases* 129 (suppl), 1974: S13–S18.

14. Meyer et al., "Plague Immunization."

15. Richard F. Platzer, "Evaluation of Therapeutic Agents in Plague," *U.S. Naval Medical Bulletin* 46, no. 11 (1946): 1676–80.

16. *AR of SSG 1900*, 21.

17. Simon Flexner, F. G. Novy, and Lewellys Barker, *Report of the Commission Appointed by the Secretary of the Treasury for the Investigation of Plague in San Francisco* (Wash., DC: GPO, 1901), 8.

18. *SFChron.*, Mar. 25, 1900; editorial, *Occidental Medical Times* 14, no. 4 (1900): 121.

19. Risse, *Plague, Fear, and Politics*, 56–59; Chase, *Barbary Plague*, 19.

20. Chase, *Barbary Plague*, 51–52.

21. Risse, *Plague, Fear, and Politics*, 123.

22. The Chinese Six Companies was an organization comprising representatives from the six districts of Guangzhou Province, where most of San Francisco's Chinese originated. They acted as a benevolent association, providing a safety net for the unemployed, settling disputes, helping with education, and the like.

23. *AR of SSG 1900*, 558–60.

24. Anon., "Society Proceedings, California Academy of Medicine: The Plague" *Occidental Medical Times* 14, no. 7 (1900): 226.

25. *SFChron.*, Jun. 11, 1900; *AR of SSG 1900*, 540.

26. One account states that about two thousand doses of vaccine were given during the Honolulu outbreak, mainly to Japanese residents. Some severe, nonfatal, side effects were noted. James C. Mohr, *Plague and Fire: Battling Black Death and the 1900 Burning of Honolulu's Chinatown* (New York: Oxford Univ. Press, 2005), 177–79. See also Meyer et al., "Plague Immunization"; and *AR of SSG 1900*, 544.

27. *AR of SSG 1900*, 22, 542–43; anon., "An Act to Prevent the Introduction of Contagious Diseases from One State to Another and for the Punishment for Certain Offenses," *Public Health Reports* 5, no. 14 (1890): 143–44.

28. Supervising Surgeon General to Station, May 22, 1900: "Department Circular No. 73, Marine Hospital Service," NARA San Bruno, RG 90, box 14, vol. 3, 1 (quotation).

29. *AR of SSG 1900*, 543–48.

30. *AR of SSG 1900*, 549.

31. *SFChron.*, Jun. 2, 1900.

32. Risse, *Plague, Fear, and Politics*, 135–39.

33. Kinyoun to Senator Cockrell, Jan. 24, 1901; Kinyoun to Bailhache, Aug. 9, 1900, Kinyoun papers, National Library of Medicine.

34. Kinyoun to Preston Bailhache, Aug. 9, 1901, Kinyoun papers.

35. Risse, *Plague, Fear, and Politics*, 140–46.

36. David M. Morens and Anthony S. Fauci, "The Forgotten Forefather: Joseph James Kinyoun and the Founding of the National Institutes of Health," *mBio* 3, no. 4 (2012), https://journals.asm.org/doi/10.1128/mBio.00139-12

37. Kinyoun to Senator Cockrell, Jan. 24, 1901, Kinyoun papers.

38. Risse, *Plague, Fear, and Politics*, 140–45.

39. Editorial, *Science* NS 13, no. 333, May 17 (1901): 761–65.

40. *AR of SSG 1901*, 495–500; quote on 499.

41. *AR of SSG 1901*, 503; Risse, *Plague, Fear, and Politics*, 176.

42. *AR of SSG 1901*, 503.

43. Esmond R. Long, *Frederick George Novy, 1864–1957: A Biographical Memoir* (Wash., DC: National Academy of Sciences, 1959), http://www.nasonline.org/publications /biographical-memoirs/memoir-pdfs/novy-frederick.pdf

44. Kalisch, "Black Death in Chinatown," 128.

45. Powel Kazanjian, "Frederick Novy and the 1901 San Francisco Plague Commission Investigation," *Clinical Infectious Diseases* 55, no. 10 (2012): 1373–78.

46. Flexner et al., *Report of the Commission*, 8.

47. Simon Flexner, "The Pathology of Bubonic Plague," *Transactions of the American Association of Physicians*, 16 (1901): 502–3.

48. Flexner et al., *Report of the Commission,* 8–9; Lewellys Barker, *Time and the Physician* (New York: Putnam, 1942), 112.

49. Lewellys Barker, "On the Clinical Aspects of Plague," *Transactions of the American Association of Physicians,* 16 (1901): 475.

50. Risse, *Plague, Fear, and Politics,* 171–73.

51. *AR of SSG 1901,* 538–40.

52. Risse, *Plague, Fear, and Politics,* 177.

53. Editorial, "The Concealment of Plague Information," *Occidental Medical Times* 15, no. 6 (1901): 215–18.

54. *AR of SSG 1901,* 538–78.

55. Various reports in *AR of SSG 1901,* 501–59; Chase, *Barbary Plague,* 107.

56. Chase, *Barbary Plague,* 91–101.

57. Anon., "Society Proceedings, California Academy of Medicine: The Plague," *Occidental Medical Times* 14, no. 7 (1900): 227.

58. *AR of SSG 1902,* 18.

59. Risse, *Plague, Fear, and Politics,* 218–22.

60. Chase, *The Barbary Plague,* 120–23.

61. Risse, *Plague, Fear, and Politics,* 254–61.

62. *AR of SG 1904,* 76, 229.

63. Risse, *Plague, Fear, and Politics,* 244–61.

CHAPTER 7. THE STATION IN MIDDLE AGE

1. *AR of SSG 1903,* 305.

2. J. M. Eager, *The Present Pandemic of Plague* (Wash., DC: GPO, 1908), 4–14.

3. *AR of SSG 1903,* 226, 237; *AR of SSG 1904,* 425–29.

4. The advisory committee was appointed by the secretary of state for India, the Royal Society, and the Lister Institute, "Experiments upon the Transmission of Plague by Fleas," *Journal of Hygiene* 6, no. 4 (1906): 425–82. *Quarantine Laws and Regulations of the United States,* rev. ed. (Wash., DC: GPO, 1903), 16.

5. *Quarantine Laws and Regulations of the United States,* rev. ed., 16.

6. Station to Surgeon General, Jul. 1, 1903, NARA San Bruno Grp. 90, box 1, 1–3; *AR of SSG 1903,* 305.

7. *AR of SSG 1902,* 353–54.

8. Myron Echenberg, *Plague Ports: The Global Urban Impact of Bubonic Plague 1894–1901* (New York: New York Univ. Press, 2007), 185–212.

9. Reynaldo C. Ileto, "Cholera and the Origins of the American Sanitary Order in the Philippines," in *Imperial Medicine and Indigenous Societies,* ed. David Arnold (New York: Manchester Univ. Press, 1988), 127; *AR of SSG 1902,* 355–8.

10. Stephen D. Coats, "Gathering at the Golden Gate: The US Army and San Francisco, 1898" (PhD diss., Univ. of Kansas, 1998), 92–93.

11. *AR of SSG 1902,* 22–24.

12. *AR of SSG 1902,* 427.

13. *AR of SSG 1902,* 368–69.

14. *AR of SSG 1900,* 640–41.

15. Surgeon General to Station, May 13, 1899, NARA San Bruno, RG 90, box 15, vol. 2.

16. *AR of SSG 1901,* 447; *AR of SSG 1902,* 349–53.

17. *AR of SSG 1901,* 476–77.

18. *AR of SSG 1905,* 188–89.

19. *AR of SSG 1902,* 427.

20. *AR of SSG 1902,* 427.

21. Surgeon General to Station, Jul. 3, 1902, NARA San Bruno, RG 90, box 24, vol. 6, 728.

22. *AR of SSG 1902,* 427.

23. Station to Surgeon General, Oct. 28, 1903, NARA San Bruno, RG 90, box 1, vol. 21, 411–13.

24. Station to Surgeon General, Jul. 1, 1903, NARA San Bruno, RG 90, box 1, vol. 21, 1–3.

25. *AR of SG 1905,* 188–89.

26. Barde, *Immigration at the Golden Gate,* 11–12.

27. Surgeon General to Station, Oct. 20, 1903, NARA San Bruno, RG 90, box 18, vol. 7.

28. See Charles E. Neu, *An Unusual Friendship: Theodore Roosevelt and Japan, 1906–1909* (Cambridge: Harvard Univ. Press, 1967), 163–80.

29. Barde, *Immigration at the Golden Gate,* 93–99.

30. MOJMHS, Sept. 20, 1901.

31. "An Act to Regulate the Immigration of Aliens into the United States," Mar. 3, 1903. *Statutes at Large of the United States of America from November, 1902 to March, 1905,* chap. 1012, 1213–22, https://tile.loc.gov/storage-services/service/ll/llsl//llsl-c57/llsl-c57.pdf; quotes on 1214.

32. *Book of Instruction for the Medical Inspection of Immigrants, Prepared by Direction of the Surgeon-General* (Wash., DC: GPO, 1903).

33. Hugh Cumming to Medical Inspector of Aliens, Surgeon F. E. Trotter, Mar. 5, 1905, NARA San Bruno, RG 90, box 2, vol. 24, 439.

34. Surgeon General to Station, Nov. 7, 1904, NARA San Bruno, RG 90, box 17, vol. 6.

35. Station to Surgeon General, Aug 11, 1903, NARA San Bruno, RG 90, box 1, vol. 21, 173.

36. *Book of Instruction for the Medical Inspection of Immigrants.*

37. Paul Tower, "The History of Trachoma: Its Military and Sociological Implications," *Archives of Ophthalmology* 69, no. 1 (1963): 123–30.

38. Shannon K. Allen and Richard D. Semba, "The Trachoma 'Menace' in the United States, 1897–1960." *Survey of Ophthalmology* 47, no. 5 (2002): 502.

39. Alan M. Kraut, *Silent Travelers: Germs, Genes, and the "Immigration Menace"* (Baltimore: Johns Hopkins Univ. Press, 1994): 66; Howard Markel, "The Eyes Have It: Trachoma, the Perception of Disease, the United States Public Health Service, and the American Jewish Immigration Experience," *Bulletin of the History of Medicine* 74, no. 3 (2000): 525–60.

40. V. Heiser to Surgeon General, Apr. 21, 1905, NARA San Bruno, RG 90, box 2, vol. 25, 236–37.

41. Surgeon General to Station, Aug. 28, 1905, NARA San Bruno, RG 90, box 18, vol. 7.

42. Station to Surgeon General, Apr. 12, 1905, NARA San Bruno, RG 90, box 2, vol. 26, 78.

43. Cumming to Immigration Commissioner, Apr. 12, 1905, NARA San Bruno, RG 90, box 2, vol. 26, 76.

44. Acting Surgeon General to Station, May 16, 1905, NARA San Bruno, RG 90, box 18, vol. 7.

45. Station to Surgeon General. May 3, 1905, NARA San Bruno, RG 90, box 2, vol. 25, 144.

46. Passed Asst. Surg. T. Clark and Passed Asst. Surg. J. W. Schereschewsky, *Trachoma: Its Character and Effects* (Wash., DC: GPO, 1907), 3–4, 13.

47. *SFChron.* Apr. 2 and Apr. 4, 1905.

48. *AR of SG 1904*, 211.

49. *AR of CGI 1911* (Wash., DC: GPO, 1912), 80–81.

50. *AR of SG 1909*, 189.

51. Shin Ji-Hye, "The 'Oriental' Problem: Trachoma and Asian Immigrants in the United States, 1897–1910," *Korean Journal of Medical History* 23, no. 3 (2014): 586–87.

52. Station to Surgeon General, May 22, 1905, NARA San Bruno, RG 90, vol. 26, 195.

53. "Trachoma among Immigrants." *New York Medical Journal* 93, no. 17 (1911): 835.

54. *SFChron.*, Aug. 4, 1905.

55. *SFChron.*, Aug. 31, 1905.

56. *Book of Instructions for the Medical Inspection of Immigrants*, 9.

57. Barde, *Immigration at the Golden Gate*, 57–75.

58. *SFChron.*, Jan. 6, 1900.

59. *SFChron.*, Sept. 9, 1908.

60. *SFChron.*, Nov. 18, 1902, 7.

61. Station to Surgeon General, Feb. 10, 1905, NARA San Bruno, RG 90, box 2, vol. 24, 394.

62. Station to Surgeon General, Nov. 9, 1905, NARA San Bruno, RG 90, box 3, vol. 30, 197.

63. *AR of SG 1901*, 487–91.

64. Station to PHMHS Hospital, Hong Kong, Sept. 30, 1909, NARA San Bruno, RG 90, box 6, vol. 38, 149–50.

65. Acting Surgeon General to Station, Apr. 30, 1909, NARA San Bruno, RG 90, box 20, vol. 12.

66. Trotter to Pacific Coast Steamship Service, Oct. 5, 1909, NARA San Bruno, RG 90, box 6, vol. 38, 167.

67. Station to Surgeon General, Jul. 24, 1903, NARA, San Bruno, RG 90, box 1, vol. 21, 88–90.

68. Station to Surgeon General, Jun. 30, 1905, NARA, San Bruno, RG 90, box 2, vol. 25, 341–44.

69. Station to Surgeon General, Jul. 5, 1907, NARA San Bruno, RG 90, box 4, vol. 32, 378–80.

70. Station to Surgeon General, Apr. 21, 1908, NARA San Bruno, RG 90, box 5, vol. 34, 432–35; quote on 433–34.

71. *AR of SSG 1899*, 822.

72. MOJMHS, Nov. 2, 1900.

73. MOJMHS, Nov. 21, 1900.

74. Station to Surgeon General, Apr. 22, 1905, NARA San Bruno, RG 90, box 2, vol. 26, 112–14.

75. Station to Surgeon General, Dec. 5, 1906 and Dec. 11, 1906, NARA San Bruno, RG 90, box 3, vol. 30, 440–42, 473–75.

76. MOJMHS, Aug. 4, 1900.

77. Station to Surgeon General, Mar. 19, 1904, NARA San Bruno, RG 90, box 2, vol. 24, 330–33; Station to Surgeon General, Dec. 23, 1904, NARA San Bruno, RG 90, box 2, vol. 24, 218.

78. Station to Surgeon General, Aug. 12, 1907, NARA San Bruno, RG 90, box 4, vol. 33, 15–16; Station to Surgeon General, Mar. 10, 1908, NARA San Bruno, RG 90, box 5, vol. 34, 306–7, 407.

79. Station to Surgeon General, Jul. 22, 1903, NARA San Bruno, RG 90, box 1, vol. 21, 78–80.

80. Station to Surgeon General, Nov. 8, 1905, NARA San Bruno, RG 90, box 3, vol. 27, 94–102; quote on 97.

81. Station to Surgeon General, Dec. 15, 1906, NARA San Bruno, RG 90, box 19, vol. 9, 485–86.

82. Station to Surgeon General, Nov. 24, 1906, NARA San Bruno, RG 90, box 3, vol. 30, 402–3; quote on 403.

83. Station to Surgeon General, Aug. 8, 1907, NARA San Bruno, RG 90, box 4, vol. 32, 486–87; quote on 486.

84. Station to Surgeon General, Jan. 18, 1906, NARA San Bruno, RG 90, box 3, vol. 28, 46–48.

85. *SFChron.*, Aug. 13, 1905.

86. Surgeon General to Station, Dec. 6, 1905, NARA San Bruno, RG 90, box 18, vol. 8.

87. Station to Surgeon General, Jun. 3, 1907, NARA San Bruno, RG 90, box 4, vol. 32, 174.

88. Station to Surgeon General, Sept. 5, 1907, NARA San Bruno, RG 90, box 4, vol. 33, 348, 350; quote on 350.

89. Station to Surgeon General, Feb. 4, 1908, NARA San Bruno, RG 90, box 5, vol. 34, 165.

CHAPTER 8. PLAGUE RETURNS

1. Andrea R. Davies, *Saving San Francisco: Relief and Recovery after the 1906 Disaster* (Philadelphia: Temple Univ. Press, 2012), 18, 26. For the earthquake and its aftermath, see also Simon Winchester, *A Crack in the Edge of the World: America and the Great California Earthquake of 1906* (New York: Harper Collins, 2005); Philip L. Fradkin, *The Great Earthquake and Firestorms of 1906: How San Francisco Nearly Destroyed Itself* (Berkeley: Univ. of California Press, 2005). There are many other works. The Museum of the City of San Francisco has an impressive amount of eyewitness information; http://www.sfmuseum.org/1906/06.html

2. The records at NARA San Bruno, CA, covering the time of the earthquake are missing. The statements about damage are based on *AR of SG 1906,* 198, and are inferred from subsequent correspondence.

3. Station to Surgeon General, Dec. 11, 1906, NARA San Bruno, RG 90, box 3, vol. 30, 473–75.

4. *SFChron.*, Dec. 11, 1906.

5. Station to Surgeon General, Mar. 11, 1907, NARA San Bruno, RG 90, box 4, vol. 31, 280–81.

6. Assistant Surgeon General to Station, Aug. 25, 1906, NARA San Bruno, RG 90, box 19, book 9.

7. *AR of SSG 1907*, 15–16, 77.

8. Station to Surgeon General, Sept. 18, 1906, NARA San Bruno, RG 90, box 3, vol. 30, 147, 156, 163–66; Station to "Agents of the Various Steamship companies & Sailing Vessels," Sept. 13, 1906, NARA San Bruno, RG 90, box 3, vol. 30, 147.

9. Station to Surgeon General, Jun. 11, 1907, NARA San Bruno, RG 90, box 4, vol. 32, 235–37.

10. This and much of the following narrative is based on Chase, *Barbary Plague*, 151–93; and Frank M. Todd, ed., *Eradicating Plague from San Francisco: Report of the Citizen's Health Committee and an Account of its Work* (San Francisco: C. A. Murdock, 1909).

11. Station to Surgeon General, Aug. 15, 1907, NARA San Bruno, RG 90, box 4, vol. 33, 26–27; quote on 27.

12. Blaisdell and Grossman, *Catastrophes, Epidemics*, 157.

13. Todd, *Eradicating Plague*, 76.

14. The rat-eradication program is summarized in *AR of SSG 1908*, 11–27. Also see Chase, *Barbary Plague*, 159–77.

15. Station to Surgeon General, Sept. 10, 1907, NARA San Bruno, RG 90, box 4, vol. 33, 155–56.

16. Hobdy to Passed Assistant Surgeon J. N. Holt, PHMHS, Columbia River, OR, NARA San Bruno, RG 90, box 4, vol. 33, 136.

17. Station to Surgeon General, Aug. 17, 1907, NARA San Bruno, RG 90, box 4, vol. 33, 47.

18. Directive issued by Angel Island Quarantine Station, Aug. 18, 1907, NARA San Bruno, RG 90, box 4, vol. 33, 48–50; quote on 48.

19. Station to Surgeon General, Aug. 17, 1907, NARA San Bruno, RG 90, box 4, vol. 33, 47.

20. Surgeon General to Station, Aug. 26, 1907, NARA San Bruno, RG 90, box 19, vol. 10.

21. Directive, Angel Island Quarantine Station, Aug. 18, 1907, NARA San Bruno, RG 90, box 4, vol. 33, 48–50.

22. *Biennial Report, California State Department of Health 1906–8*, 15–18.

23. Station to Surgeon General, Sept. 11, 1907, NARA San Bruno, RG 90, box 4, vol. 33, 159–63.

24. Station to Surgeon General, Sept. 17, 1907, NARA San Bruno, RG 90, box 4, vol. 33, 179–83; quote on 183.

25. Surgeon General to Station, Sept. 24, 1907, NARA San Bruno, RG 90, box 19, vol. 9.

26. Station to Surgeon General, Oct. 1, 1907, NARA San Bruno, RG 90, box 4, vol. 33, 252–54.

27. *AR of SSG 1908*, 31–33.

28. Surgeon General to Station, Nov. 2, 1907, NARA San Bruno, RG 90, box 19, vol. 10.

29. Station to Surgeon General, Oct. 11, 1907, NARA San Bruno, RG 90, box 4, vol. 33, 298–300, 310; quote on 299.

30. Station to Secretary, CSBH (N. K. Foster), Oct. 21, 1907, NARA San Bruno, RG 90, box 4, vol. 33, 311–13; quote on 313.

31. Station to Surgeon General, Oct. 22, 1907, NARA San Bruno, RG 90, box 4, vol. 33, 317.

32. Station to Surgeon General, Oct. 22 and 30, 1907, NARA San Bruno, RG 90, box 4, vol. 33, 317–18 and 348–50.

33. Station to Surgeon General, Sept. 5, 1907, NARA San Bruno, RG 90, box 4, vol. 33, 396.

34. Station to Surgeon General, May 22, 1908, NARA San Bruno, RG 90, box 5, vol. 35, 48–49; *SFMo.*, May 20, 1908.

35. Station to Surgeon General, Feb. 11, 1908, NARA San Bruno, RG 90, box 5, vol. 34; 186–87.

36. Station to Surgeon General, Apr. 25, 1908, NARA San Bruno, RG 90, box 5, vol. 34, 469–78.

37. Station to Surgeon General, Jan. 2, 1908, NARA San Bruno, RG 90, box 5, vol. 34, 40–41.

38. Station to Surgeon General, Feb. 1, 1908, NARA San Bruno, RG 90, box 5, vol. 34, 152–53.

39. *AR of SSG 1908*, 34–39.

40. Station to Surgeon General, Feb. 28, 1908, NARA San Bruno, RG 90, box 5, vol. 34, 250–57; Station to Surgeon General, Mar. 10, 1908, NARA San Bruno, RG 90, box 5, vol. 34, 303–4.

41. Station to Surgeon General, Feb. 26, 1907, NARA San Bruno, RG 90, box 4, vol. 31, 261.

42. *AR of SSG 1914*, 142.

43. Hobdy to Passed Assistant Surgeon John N. Holt, Feb. 1, 1908, NARA San Bruno, RG 90, box 5, vol. 34, 152–53.

44. *AR of SSG 1908*, 24. Todd, *Eradicating Plague*, 183, gives a total of 160 cases.

45. Station to Surgeon General, Jun. 5, 1908, NARA San Bruno, RG 90, box 5, vol. 35, 84.

46. Station to Surgeon General, Oct. 24, 1908, NARA San Bruno, RG 90, box 5, vol. 36, 204.

47. *AR of SSG 1909*, 11.

CHAPTER 9. FULL MATURITY AND IMMIGRATION

1. Map of San Francisco Quarantine Station, February 1913, NARA College Park, RG 90, box 42, folder #3, 05119–0245 to 0315; List of Buildings at San Francisco quarantine station, Jul. 6, 1915, NARA College Park, RG 90, box 42, folder #3, 05119–0245; Report of Inspection of the quarantine station, Oct. 16, 1916 (erroneously noted as 1906 on the report), NARA College Park, RG 90, box 42, folder 1850–15.

2. Status report, estimate for improvements, date not given but 1917 or 1918 based on dates in report, NARA College Park, RG 90, box 42, folder 0750–235.

3. Station to Surgeon General, Jan. 5, 1914, NARA San Bruno, RG 90, box 8, vol. B2, 378–79, 391–92.

4. Station to Surgeon General, Jan. 8, 1913, NARA San Bruno, RG 90, box 7, vol. 43, 424–25; quote on 424.

5. Station to Surgeon General, Jun. 11, 1918, NARA San Bruno, RG 90, box 9, vol. B6, 27.

6. Station to Surgeon General, May 21, 1923, NARA San Bruno, RG 90, box 11, vol. 11.

7. Station to Surgeon General, Jul. 12, 1924, NARA San Bruno, RG 90, box 12, vol. 13, 41–49; Station to Surgeon General, Jun. 6, 1923, NARA College Park, RG 90, box 44, folder 1975–270; Station to Surgeon General, Oct. 11, 1922, NARA San Bruno, RG 90, box 11, vol. 10, 313.

8. Station to Surgeon General, May 16, 1914, NARA San Bruno, RG 90, box 8, vol. B3, 32–33.

9. Station to Surgeon General, Nov. 3, 1913, NARA San Bruno, RG 90, box 8, vol. 32, 247–48.

10. Report of repairs and improvements during the fiscal year ended Jun. 30, 1917, NARA San Bruno, RG 90, box 9, vol. B5, 105.

11. Station to Surgeon General, Sept. 3, 1913, NARA San Bruno, RG 90, box 8, vol. B2, 246–49.

12. Station to Surgeon General, Apr. 5, 1921, NARA San Bruno, RG 90, box 10, vol. B8, 485.

13. Station to Surgeon General, Jun. 12, 1913, NARA San Bruno, RG 90, box 8, vol. B2, 115–18.

14. Station to Surgeon General, Sept. 8, 1920, NARA San Bruno, RG 90, box 10, vol. B8, 248–54.

15. Station to Surgeon General, May 20, 1923, NARA San Bruno, RG 90, box 11, vol. 11; quote on 2 of letter.

16. Station to Surgeon General, Jun. 30, 1910, NARA San Bruno CA, RG 90, box 8, vol. 39, 317–19.

17. Station to Surgeon General, Feb. 3, 1913, NARA San Bruno, RG 90, box 7, vol. 43, 458–60; quote on 460.

18. Station to Secretary, CSBH, Mar. 29, 1910, NARA San Bruno, RG 90, box 6, vol. 39, 32–34; Station to Supervising Architect, Treasury Dept., Mar. 31, 1910, box 6, vol. 39, 42–43; Station to Surgeon General, Apr. 4, 1910, box 6, vol. 39, 49–57; Station to Surgeon General, Jul. 19, 1910, box 6, vol. 39, 390–92; Since the Navy insisted on mandatory vaccination on entry to the Navy, Trotter speculated that those with smallpox or without vaccination scars had either received faulty lymph or had wiped off the material before it had a chance to take. Station to Surgeon General, Mar. 29, 1910, NARA San Bruno, RG 90, box 6, vol. 39, 32–34.

19. *AR of SG 1920*, 150–51.

20. Station to W. H. Avery, Toyo Kisen Kaisha, San Francisco, May 5, 1910, NARA San Bruno, RG 90, box 6, vol. 39, 121–12; Station to Mr. R. P. Schwerin, PMSS, San Francisco, May 4, 1910, NARA San Bruno, RG 90, box 6, vol. 39, 123–25; Station to Mr. Frey, assistant manager, PMSS, May 30, 1910, NARA San Bruno, RG 90, box 6, vol. 39, 187–88.

21. *AR of SG 1915*, 149.

22. Station to Surgeon General, Jul. 10, 1917, NARA College Park, RG 90, box 42, folder 1850–15.

23. Station to Passed Assistant Carl Ramus, Territory of Hawaii, Jun. 21, 1910, NARA San Bruno, RG 90, box 6, vol. 39, 278–79.

24. Leland E. Cofer, "Maritime Quarantine," *Public Health Bulletin No. 34* (Wash., DC: GPO, 1910), 35.

25. Station to Surgeon General, Jul. 10, 1917, NARA College Park, RG 90, box 42, folder 1850–15.

26. Pollitzer, *Cholera*, 865–73.

27. Erika Lee and Judy Yung, *Angel Island: Immigrant Gateway to America* (New York: Oxford Univ. Press, 2010), 12–15, 36–38.

28. *AR of SG 1921,* 235.

29. The numerous problems are detailed in Toogood, *A Civil History*, 378–429.

30. *Immigration Act,* 1891, Records of 51st Congress, Sess. 2, 1891, chap 551.

31. The PHMHS was renamed the Public Health Service in 1912 and retains that name today.

32. Bailey K. Ashford and Pedro Gutierrez Igaravidez, "Summary of a Ten Year's Campaign against Hookworm in Porto Rico," *JAMA* 54, no. 22 (1910): 1757–61.

33. Charles Wardell Stiles, "A Brief Review of Certain Phases of Hookworm Disease," in *Transactions of the Seventh Annual Conference of State and Territorial Health Officers with the United States Public Health and Marine-Hospital Service, June 2, 1909* (Wash., DC: GPO, 1910), 59–62.

34. *Book of Instructions for the Medical Inspection of Aliens (Revised Jan. 18, 1910)* (Wash., DC: GPO, 1910), 9.

35. *AR of CGI 1912* (Wash., DC: GPO), 120–21; *AR of CGI 1917,* 120–21; *AR of CGI 1921,* 130–31.

36. Toogood, *A Civil History*, 382; Nayan Shah, *Contagious Divides: Epidemics and Race in San Francisco's Chinatown* (Berkeley: Univ. of California Press, 2001), 190–92.

37. *AR of SG 1912,* 142–43.

38. *AR of SG 1912,* 142–44; *AR of SG 1915,* 211–12; *AR of SG 1916,* 226–27.

39. *AR of SG, 1913,* 162–63.

40. *AR of SG, 1914,* 221–23.

41. Bureau of Immigration to Surgeon General, Mar. 18, 1919, and accompanying regulations, NARA College Park, RG 90, box 42, folder 0425–183; *Regulations Governing the Medical Inspection of Aliens* (Washington, DC: GPO, 1917).

42. Lee and Yung, *Angel Island,* 39.

43. *AR of SG 1917,* 184–85; *AR of SG 1918,* 257–58; *AR of SG 1928,* 171; N. E. Wayson, "Clonorchis Investigations: A Summary of Surveys and Experiments to Determine Whether Clonorchiasis may be Disseminated in the Pacific Slope of the United States," *Public Health Reports* 42, no. 51 (1927): 3129–35; Yu Fong Wong, *Historical Review of Clonorchiasis* (San Francisco: Chinese Six Companies, 1927).

44. "An Act to Regulate the Immigration of Aliens to, and the Residence of Aliens in, the United States," Record of 64th Congress, Sess. 2, chap 29, Feb. 5, 1917, Sec. 16, https://curiosity.lib.harvard.edu/immigration-to-the-united-states-1789-1930/catalog /39-990100032410203941

45. *AR of SG 1920,* 173–74.

46. H. M. Lai, "Island of Immortals: Chinese Immigrants and the Angel Island Immigration Station," *California History* 57, no. 1 (1978): 88–103; *SFChron.,* Nov. 1, 1922; quote on 8. There is also a large body of literature, including personal memoirs, on life in the Immigration Station. The details, however, are beyond the scope of this book.

47. For details see Sarah J. Moore, *Empire on Display: San Francisco's Panama-Pacific International Exposition of 1915* (Norman: Univ. of Oklahoma Press, 2013), 97–132.

48. *SFChron.*, Oct. 7, 1919.

49. An excellent account of the epidemic, prepared by the University of Michigan Center for the History of Medicine, can be seen at http://www.influenzaarchive.org/cities /city-sanfrancisco.html#

50. *SFChron.*, Oct. 26, 1918.

51. *SFChron.*, Nov. 9, 1918.

52. Arnold Woods, "Spanish Flu in SF: A Closer Look," *Open SF History*, Mar. 2020, https://opensfhistory.org/news/2020/03/14/spanish-flu-in-sf-a-closer-look/

53. M. W. Ireland and F. W. Weed, *The Medical Department of the United States Army in the World War, Volume 5: Military Hospitals in the United States* (Wash., DC: GPO, 1923), 492.

54. *SFChron.*, Nov. 9, 1918.

55. Station to Surgeon General, Nov. 21, 1918, NARA San Bruno, RG 90, box 9, vol. 6, 294.

56. Station to Surgeon General, Nov. 21, 1918, NARA San Bruno CA, RG 90, box 9, vol. 6, 328–29; Station to Surgeon General, Nov. 21, 1918, NARA San Bruno CA, RG 90. box 9, vol. 6, 407, 437.

57. *AR of SG 1920*, 124.

58. *AR of SG 1919*, 113.

59. L. E. Cofer, "A Word to Ship Captains about Quarantine: An Open Letter to Ship Captains," *Public Health Bulletin* No. 55 (Wash., DC: GPO, Jul. 1912), 1–15.

CHAPTER 10. THE CYANIDE ERA

1. For details, see Lien-the Wu, *Plague Fighter: The Autobiography of a Modern Chinese Physician* (Cambridge, XX: W. Heffer, 1959); and William Summers, *The Great Manchurian Plague of 1910–1911: The Geopolitics of an Epidemic Disease* (New Haven, CT: Yale Univ. Press, 2012).

2. Harrison, *Contagion*, 201–3.

3. *AR of SG 1910*, 143–51; *AR of SG 1911*, 182–88.

4. *AR of SG 1910*, 83.

5. Station to Surgeon General, Jun. 18, 1910, NARA San Bruno, RG 90, box 6, vol. 39, 269–71; *AR of SG 1915*, 139.

6. Station to Surgeon General, Sept. 17, 1910, NARA San Bruno, RG 90, box 7, vol. 40, 85–87; Surgeon General to Station, Sept. 30, 1910, NARA San Bruno, RG 90. box 20, vol. 12.

7. *Quarantine Laws and Regulation of the United States*, rev. ed. (Wash., DC: GPO, 1910), 39; *AR of SG 1911*, 120–21; quote on 121.

8. Surgeon General to Station, Apr. 5 and Apr. 25, 1911, NARA, San Bruno RG 90, box 20, vol. 12.

9. Charles Chapin, "The Fetish of Disinfection," *JAMA* 47, no. 8 (1906): 574–80; Charles Chapin, *The Sources and Modes of Infection*, 2nd ed. (New York: John Wiley, 1916), 164–212.

10. Station to Surgeon General, Jun. 30, 1912, NARA, San Bruno, RG 90, box 7, vol. 43, 116–17, 154–56, 165–66.

11. Surgeon General to Station, Jul. 26, 1912, NARA San Bruno, RG 90, box 21, vol. 14; Station to Surgeon General, Jul. 16, 1912, NARA San Bruno, RG 90. box 8, vol. B1, 154–56.

12. R. H. Creel, "The Extension of Plague Infection of the Bubonic Type," *American Journal of Public Health* 6, no. 3 (1916): 191–221.

13. *AR of SG 1915*, 223; Vernon B. Link, "The New Orleans Epidemics," chap. 5 in *A History of Plague in the United States of America*, Public Health Monograph #26 (Wash., DC: GPO, 1955), 48.

14. *Annual Report California State Board of Horticulture 1890* (Sacramento: State Printing Office, 1890), 351–52; Walter Reuther, E. Clair Calavan, and Glenn E. Carman, eds., *The Citrus Industry*, vol. 5 (Oakland: Division of Agriculture and Natural Resources, Univ. of California, 1989), 295.

15. *Hearings on General Tariff Revision Before the Committee on Ways and Means, House of Representatives*, Part 5 (Wash., DC: GPO, 1921), 3986.

16. *Quarantine Laws and Regulations of the United States, Revised Edition: October 1910 (Wash., DC: GPO, 1910)*, 52.

17. *AR of SG 1913*, 104–5.

18. *AR of SG 1915*, 213–44; Link, "New Orleans Epidemics," 43–53.

19. "U.S. Public Health Service Bureau Circular No. 79," Oct. 30, 1915, 61–62; and "U.S. Public Health Service Bureau Circular No. 100," Nov. 4, 1916, 78–79; both in *Bureau Circular Letters, 1913–1920* (Wash., DC: GPO, 1921)

20. "U.S. Public Health Service Bureau Circular No. 100," 78–79.

21. N. Roberts, "Fumigation of the USS *Tennessee* by the Cyanide Method," *United States Naval Medical Bulletin*, 10, no. 2 (1916): 299.

22. Station to Surgeon General, Jun. 30, 1913. NARA, San Bruno, RG 90, box 8, vol. B2, 156–57; Station to Surgeon General, Apr. 28, 1914, NARA, San Bruno, RG 90, box 8, vol. B3, 10–11.

23. Rupert Blue, "Fumigation of Vessels to Prevent the Spread of Plague," *Public Health Reports* 28, no. 8 (1913): 346–47.

24. Station to Surgeon General, Sept. 3, 1913, NARA, San Bruno, RG 90, box 8, vol. B2, 248–49.

25. Station to Surgeon General, Jun. 30, 1914, NARA, San Bruno, RG 90, box 8, vol. B3, 109–11.

26. Assistant Surgeon General to Station, and reply, Jan. 14, 1916, and Mar. 7, 1916, NARA, San Bruno, RG 90, box 8, vol. B3, 46.

27. *AR of SG 1916*, 119.

28. Station to Surgeon General, Mar. 23, 1916, NARA, San Bruno, RG 90, box 8, vol. B3, 57–59.

29. *Public Health Reports* 46, no. 29 (1931): 1682.

30. *AR of SG 1916*, 141–42.

31. Station to Surgeon General, Jul. 13, 1916, NARA, San Bruno, RG 90, box 9, vol. B4, 162–64.

32. Station to Surgeon General, Aug. 2, 1918, NARA College Park, box 45, folder 2210–68, "fumigations."

33. Station to Surgeon General, NARA San Bruno, RG 90, box 10, vol. B8, 257–64; Roessler & Hasslacher Chemical Company to Acting Surgeon General, Sept. 17, 1920,

NARA College Park, RG 90, box 43, folder 1975–68; Station to Surgeon General, Sept. 20, 1920, NARA College Park, RG 90, box 43, folder 1975–68.

34. *AR of SG 1916*, 142.

35. *SFChron.*, Oct. 9, 1916.

36. State of California Coroner's Inquisition, Oct. 23, 1916, NARA College Park, RG 90, box 45, folder 2210–68, Fumigations, no. 5396; all quotations from this one-page coroner's report.

37. *AR of SG 1917*, 85.

38. Station to Surgeon General, Jul. 13, 1916, NARA College Park, RG 90, folder 1850–15, #5396.

39. Station to Surgeon General, Nov. 9, 1916, NARA, San Bruno, RG 90, box 9, vol. B4, 304–6.

40. *SFChron.*, Nov. 4, 5, and 18, 1916; quote is in Coroner's Report, *SFMR*, 1917, 958.

41. Assistant Surgeon General to Medical Officer in Charge, Nov. 17, 1916, NARA San Bruno, RG 90, box 22, vol. 16.

42. Station to Surgeon General, Mar. 28, 1921, NARA San Bruno, RG 90, box 10, vol. B8, 473; 475–76.

43. Station to Surgeon General, Oct. 9, 1919, NARA San Bruno, RG 90, box 10, vol. B7, 295–96; quote on 296.

44. Station to Surgeon General, Jul. 15, 1919, NARA San Bruno, RG 90, box 10, vol. B7, 172–78.

45. Station to Surgeon General, Oct. 23, 1919, NARA San Bruno, RG 90, box 10, vol. B7, 332–35.

46. *AR of SG 1920*, 151.

47. Station to Surgeon General, Jun. 11, 1920, NARA College Park, RG 90, box 45, folder 2210–68, "fumigations."

48. *AR of SG 1922*, 165–68.

49. Station to Surgeon General, Aug. 1, 1921, NARA College Park, RG 90, box 45, folder 2210–68, "fumigations 1981"; Station to Surgeon General, Aug. 9, 1921, NARA San Bruno, RG 90, box 10, vol. B9, 127–28.

50. Station to James Whitmore, Surveyor General of Real Estate, Treasury Dept. Sept. 21, 1921, NARA College Park, RG 90, box 42, folder 05119-0315; Station to Surgeon General, Dec. 8, 1921, NARA College Park, RG 90, box 43, folder 1975–69, no. 3352.

51. Cyanide Fumigation Company to Surgeon General, Aug. 8, 1921, NARA College Park, RG 90, box 45, folder 2210–68, "fumigations 1981."

52. Station to Surgeon General, Dec. 24, 1921, NARA San Bruno, RG 90, box 10, vol. B9, 310–15.

53. Station to Surgeon General, Mar. 3, 1922, NARA San Bruno, RG 90, box 10, vol. B9, 427–43; Station to Surgeon General, Mar. 10, 1922, NARA San Bruno, RG 90, box 10, vol. B9, 457–61; *SFChron.*, Mar. 1, 1922.

54. Station to Surgeon General, Mar. 22, 1922, NARA San Bruno, RG 90, box 10, vol. B9, 478–80; Coroner, City and County of San Francisco, to Station, Apr. 11, 1922, NARA College Park, box 45, folder 2210-68/5396 (Jury verdict is on a one page insert).

55. R. H. Creel to Friench Simpson, Apr. 28, 1922, NARA College Park, RG 90, box 45, folder 2210-68/5396.

56. Station to Surgeon General, Mar. 10, 1922, NARA San Bruno, RG 90, box 11, vol. 10, 36–44; quote on 41.

57. J. G. Perry, Senior Surgeon, Public Health Service to Surgeon General, May 17, 1922, NARA College Park, RG 90, box 45, folder 2210-68/5396.

58. Station to Surgeon General, Aug. 17, 1922, NARA San Bruno, RG 90, box 11, vol. 10, 238; *AR of SG 1923*, 138–39.

59. Station to Surgeon General, Sept. 29, 1922, NARA San Bruno, RG 90, box 11, vol. B10, 291–303.

60. Station to Surgeon General, Sept. 27, 1922, NARA, San Bruno, RG 90, box 11, vol. 10, 263–75; *SFChron.*, Sept. 16, 1922.

61. Station to Surgeon General, Sept. 29, 1922, NARA San Bruno, RG 90, box 11, vol. 10, 311–19.

62. Station to Surgeon General, Sept. 29, 1922, NARA San Bruno, RG 90, box 11, vol. 10, 295–303; quote on 302.

63. Station to Assistant Surgeon General, Dec. 12, 1922, NARA San Bruno, RG 90, box 11, vol. 10, 448–51; Station to Assistant Surgeon General, Sept. 29, 1922, NARA College Park, RG 90, box 45, folder 2210-68/5396.

64. Station to Surgeon General, Dec. 18, 1922, NARA San Bruno, RG 90, box 11, vol. 10, 471–73; Station to Surgeon General, Nov. 7, 1923, NARA College Park, RG 90, box 43, folder 1850-15.

65. Station to Surgeon General, Feb. 15, 1923, NARA College Par, RG90, box 43, folder 15119.

66. Station to Surgeon General, Sept. 29, 1922, NARA San Bruno, RG 90, box 11, vol. 10, 291.

67. Station to Surgeon General, Nov. 15, 1922, NARA San Bruno, RG 90, box 11, vol. 10, 397–98.

68. "Ship Fumigation: Preliminary Report of the Board Appointed by the Surgeon General to Investigate the Subject of Fumigation of Ships," *Public Health Reports* 37, no. 44 (1922): 2744–47.

69. Station to Surgeon General, Feb. 13, 1923, NARA San Bruno, RG 90, box 11, vol. 11.

70. Station to Surgeon L. R. Thompson, Apr. 14, 1923, NARA College Park, RG 90, box 45, folder 2210–68; Station to Public Health Service, Apr. 14, 1923, NARA College Park, RG 90, box 45, folder 2210–68, "fumigations 1923"; Station to Surgeon General, Feb. 15, 1923, NARA College Park, RG 90, box 43, folder 1975–68.

71. "Cyanogen Chloride Gas Mixture: Irritating Quality of New Fumigant Saves the Life of a Stowaway on Vessel Being Fumigated," *Public Health Reports* 39, no. 11 (1924): 529.

72. Station to Surgeon General, May 21, 1923, NARA College Park, RG 90, box 45, folder 2210–68, "fumigations 1923."

73. Station to Surgeon General, Oct. 20, 1923, NARA San Bruno, RG 90, box 11, vol. 12.

74. Station to Surgeon General, Jun. 27, NARA San Bruno, RG 90, box 11, vol. 11; quote on 2.

75. Station to Surgeon General, Aug. 25, 1923, NARA San Bruno, RG 90, box 11, vol. 11.

76. J. R. Ridlon, "Some Aspects of Ship Fumigation," *Public Health Reports* 46, no. 27 (1931): 1572–78.

77. *AR of SG 1927,* 129–30.

78. *AR of SG 1928,* 128–32, 148–50.

79. *AR of SG 1921,* 190.

CHAPTER II. FINAL YEARS

1. *AR of SG 1927,* 186–90.

2. *AR of SG 1931,* 152–53.

3. *Biennial Report of the Department of Public Health of California FY 1930–2,* 40; *Biennial Report of the Department of Public Health of California FY 1934–36,* 31.

4. Kevin Starr, *Golden Gate: The Life and Times of America's Greatest Bridge* (New York: Bloomsbury Press, 2010), 109–36.

5. John C. Ralston, *This Date in San Francisco: 366 Days in the History of our Beloved Fascinating City* (Mountain View, CA: RIW Publishing, 2011), 268–69.

6. These figures are from *AR of SG* for the respective fiscal years.

7. *SFChron.,* Oct. 14, 1930.

8. Station to Surgeon General, Oct. 14, 1919, NARA San Bruno, RG 90, box 10, vol. B7, 307–8.

9. Station to Surgeon General, Mar. 28, 1944, NARA College Park, RG 90, box 14, folder 1960.

10. *AR of SG 1929,* 117–18.

11. Gerald L. Mandell, John E. Bennett, and Raphael Dolin, *Principles and Practice of Infectious Diseases,* 5th ed (Philadelphia: Churchill Livingstone, 2000), 961–92.

12. Morton N. Swartz, "Bacterial Meningitis—A View of the Past 90 Years," *New England Journal of Medicine* 351(18), 2004: 1826–87.

13. *AR of SG 1929,* 139–40.

14. *AR of SG 1930,* 134–35, 155–56.

15. *AR of SG 1930,* 68–69; K. F. Meyer, "The Ecology of Psittacosis and Ornithosis," *Medicine* 21(2), 1942: 175–206.

16. *AR of SG 1930,* 135–36.

17. Secretary of War to Secretary of Treasury, Dec. 28, 1936, NARA College Park, RG 90, box 14, file 1960-175; quote in this one-page letter.

18. Secretary of War to Secretary of Treasury, May 29, 1937, NARA College Park, RG 90, box 14, file 1960-175.

19. Station to Surgeon General, Jun. 23, 1942, NARA College Park, RG 90, box 14, folder 1850.

20. L. F. Lucaccini, "The Public Health Service on Angel Island," *Public Health Reports* 111, no. 1 (1996): 92–94.

21. "San Francisco Quarantine Station Annual Report for the Fiscal Year Ending Jun. 1937," NARA College Park, RG 90, box 14, file 1850-15.

22. *SFChron.,* Sept. 30, 1937; *SFChron.,* Jul. 30, 1940.

23. Station to Surgeon General, Jul. 15, 1936, NARA College Park, RG 90, box 14, file 1850-15.

24. Station to FQD, Aug. 11 and Oct. 25, 1938, NARA College Park, RG 90, box 14, file 1960.

25. *AR of SG 1939*, 1.

26. *SFChron.*, Apr. 11, 1940.

27. *New York Times*, Dec. 20 and Dec. 21, 1939.

28. *SFChron.*, Jan. 19, 1940.

29. Station to FQD, Jul. 4, 1940, NARA College Park, RG90, box 14, file 1850.

30. *SFChron.*, Mar. 6, 1940.

31. *SFChron.*, Aug. 13, 1940.

32. *SFChron.*, Sept. 18, 1940.

33. *SFChron.*, Mar. 18, 1941; The episode is also summarized in Lee and Yung, *Angel Island*, 299–302.

34. *SFChron.*, Jan. 28 and Mar. 14, 1941.

35. *SFChron.*, Jun. 1, 1941.

36. Station to Surgeon General, Jun. 23, 1942, NARA College Park, RG 90, box 14, folder 1850.

37. Station to Surgeon General, Jul. 7, 1942, NARA, College Park, RG 90, box 14, folder 1850.

38. *AR of SG 1942*, 7; *SFChron.*, Apr. 24, 1941.

39. *AR of SG 1942*, 8.

40. Station to Surgeon General, Aug. 6, 1942, NARA College Park, RG 90, box 14, folder 1616.

41. Station to Surgeon General, Aug. 6, 1942, NARA, College Park, RG 90, box 14, folder 1616.

42. Station to Surgeon General, Dec. 9, 10, and 18, 1942, NARA, College Park, RG 90, box 14, folder 1416.

43. *SFChron.*, Jun. 13 and Jun. 15, 1943.

44. *SFChron.*, Aug. 29, 1946.

45. *SFChron.*, Jul. 13, 1946.

46. *SFChron.*, Oct. 18, 1946.

47. *SFChron.*, Nov. 27, 1948.

48. *SFChron.*, Jan. 10, 1949; *SFChron.*, Mar. 11, 1954.

CHAPTER 12. EPILOGUE

1. Anon., "Milton Joseph Rosenau," *American Journal of Public Health*, 36 no. 5 (1936): 530–31.

2. Office of the Surgeon General, US Department of Health and Human Services, https://web.archive.org/web/20080916014409/http://surgeongeneral.gov/about/previous/bioblue.htm

3. "The Tuskegee Timeline," Centers for Disease Control and Prevention, https://www.cdc.gov/tuskegee/timeline.htm

4. "Hugh Smith Cumming (1920–1936)," Surgeon General Website, http://wayback.archive-it.org/3929/20171201191738/https://www.surgeongeneral.gov/about/previous/biocumming.html

5. *Pacific Commercial Advertiser*, Nov. 16, 1909; *Honolulu Star-Bulletin*, Nov. 10, 1917; *Oakland Tribune*, Dec. 29, 1938.

6. This is *Trypanosoma evansi,* the cause of surra, a fatal disease of horses and other animals in Africa, Asia, and South America.

7. Morens and Fauci, "The Forgotten Forefather."

8. Anon. "Dr. Walter Wyman," *Journal of the American Public Health Association* 1, no. 12 (1911): 869–70; "Walter Wyman (1891–1911," Surgeon General Website, at http://wayback .archive-it.org/3929/20171201191736/https://www.surgeongeneral.gov/about/previous /biowyman.html

9. All statements about current quarantine practices can be found at the Centers for Disease Control and Prevention website.

Bibliography

ARCHIVAL SOURCES

Annual Report of the California State Board of Horticulture. Sacramento: State Printing Office, 1890.

Appendix to the Journals of the Senate and Assembly of the Twenty-Sixth Session of the Legislature of the State of California. Sacramento: J. D. Young, Superintendent of State Printing, 1889.

Bureau Circular Letters, 1913–1920. Washington, DC: Government Printing Office, 1921.

Bureau Circulars. Washington, DC: US Department of the Treasury.

General Statutes of the State of California. Sacramento: J. D. Young, Superintendent of State Printing.

Hearings on General Tariff Revision before the Committee on Ways and Means, House of Representatives. Part 5. Washington, DC: Government Printing Office, 1921.

Immigration Act, 1891. Records of Fifty-First Congress, Session 2, 1891. Washington, DC: Government Printing Office.

Medical Officer's Journal, Angel Island Quarantine Station. Located at Maritime Research Center, San Francisco, Maritime National Historical Park. (The log books are not published, but are hand-written records. The dates covered are June 15, 1891, to November 17, 1903.)

Quarantine Laws and Regulations. February 24, 1893. US Department of the Treasury. Washington, DC: Government Printing Office, 1893.

Quarantine Laws and Regulations of the United States, rev. ed. Washington, DC: Government Printing Office, 1903.

Quarantine Laws and Regulations of the United States, rev. ed. Washington, DC: Government Printing Office, 1910.

Statutes of California Passed at the First Session of the Legislature. Sacramento CA, 1850.

US National Archives and Records Administration, Record Group 90, San Bruno, CA.

US National Archives and Records Administration, Record Group 90, College Park, MD.

Health Department Reports

Annual Report of National Board of Health. Washington, DC: Government Printing Office, 1880–85.

Annual Report of the Board of Health to the General Assembly of Louisiana. New Orleans: Board of Health, 1875–84.

Annual Report of the San Francisco Department of Health. San Francisco: San Francisco Department of Public Health, 1876–1904.

Annual Report of the Supervising Surgeon General of the Marine Hospital Service of the United States. Washington, DC: Government Printing Office, 1884–1901.

Annual Report of the Surgeon General of the Public Health and Marine Hospital Service of the United States. Washington, DC: Government Printing Office, 1902–11.

Annual Report of the Surgeon General of the Public Health Service of the United States. Washington, DC: Government Printing Office, 1912–30.

Biennial Report of the Louisiana State Board of Health. Baton Rouge: Louisiana State Board of Health, 1885–89.

Biennial Report of the State Board of Health of California (after 1925: *Biennial Report of the Department of Public Health of California*). Sacramento: California State Board of Health, 1870–1908.

Bureau Circular Letters. U.S. Treasury Department. Washington, DC: Government Printing Office, 1913–1920.

"Health Officer's Reports." *San Francisco Municipal Reports.* San Francisco: Board of Supervisors, 1865–1917.

Papers

Kinyoun Papers, National Library of Medicine.

Newspapers

Albuquerque Morning Democrat
Daily Alta California
Los Angeles Times
New Orleans Daily Picayune
New York Herald
New York Times
San Francisco Chronicle
San Francisco Examiner
San Francisco Morning Call

Compilations

American National Biography. New York: Oxford Univ. Press, 1999.

Dissertations and Theses

Coats, Stephen D. "Gathering at the Golden Gate: The U.S. Army and San Francisco, 1898." PhD diss., Univ. of Kansas, 1998.

Shah, Nyan. "San Francisco's Chinatown: Race and Cultural Politics of Public Health, 1854–1952." PhD diss., Univ. of Michigan, 1995.

Skubik, Mark M. "Public Health Politics and the San Francisco Plague Epidemic of 1900–1904." Master's thesis, San Jose State Univ., 2002.

PUBLISHED DOCUMENTS

"A Brief Review of Certain Phases of Hookworm Disease." *Transactions of the Seventh Annual Conference of State and Territorial Health Officers with the United States Public*

Health and Marine-Hospital Service, Jun. 2, 1909, Washington, DC: Government Printing Office, 1910: 59–64.

Advisory Committee, appointed by the Secretary of State for India, the Royal Society, and the Lister Institute. "Experiments upon the Transmission of Plague by Fleas." *Journal of Hygiene* 6, no. 4 (1906): 425–82.

Allen, Shannon K., and Richard D. Semba. "The Trachoma 'Menace' in the United States, 1897–1960." *Survey of Ophthalmology* 47, no. 5 (2002): 500–509.

Anonymous. "An Act to Prevent the Introduction of Contagious Diseases from One State to Another and for the Punishment for Certain Offenses." *Public Health Reports* 5, no. 14 (1890): 143–44.

Anonymous. "Dr. Hamilton Resigns—Says he has been Driven out of Office by Surgeon-General Wyman." *Indiana Medical Journal* 15, no. 5 (1896): 179–80.

Anonymous. "In Honor of Dr. Joseph J. Kinyoun, U. S. Marine Hospital Service." *Georgetown College Journal* 27, no. 9 (1899): 420–22.

Anonymous. "Louisiana Quarantine." *Journal of the American Medical Association* 21, no. 18 (1893): 662–63.

Anonymous. "Quarantine at New York." *Harper's Weekly* 23, no. 1184 (Sept. 6, 1879): 706.

Anonymous. "Society Proceedings, California Academy of Medicine: The Plague." *Occidental Medical Times* 14, no. 7 (1900): 220–27.

Anonymous. "The Quarantine Station at San Francisco." *Occidental Medical Times* 3, no. 1 (1889): 34–36.

Ashford, Bailey K., and Pedro Gutierrex Igaravidez. "Summary of a Ten Year's Campaign against Hookworm in Porto Rico." *Journal of the American Medical Association* 54, no. 22 (1910): 1757–61.

Atkinson, William B., ed. *The Physicians and Surgeons of the United States.* Philadelphia: Charles Robson, 1878.

Baldwin, Peter. *Contagion and the State in Europe.* Cambridge: Cambridge Univ. Press, 1999.

Barde, Robert E. *Immigration at the Golden Gate: Passenger Ships, Exclusion, and Angel Island.* Westport, CT: Praeger, 2008.

Barde, Robert. "Prelude to the Plague: Public Health and Politics at America's Pacific Gateway, 1899." *Journal of the History of Medicine* 58, no. 3 (2003): 153–86.

Barker, Lewellys. "On the Clinical Aspects of Plague." *Transactions of the American Association of Physicians* 16, 1901: 459–80.

Barker, Lewellys. *Time and the Physician.* New York: Putnam, 1942.

Barua, Dhiman. "History of Cholera." In *Cholera*, edited by Dhiman Barua and William B. Greenough III. New York: Springer, 1992, 1–7.

Blaisdell, F. William, and Moses Grossman. *Catastrophes, Epidemics, and Neglected Diseases: San Francisco General Hospital and the Evolution of Public Care.* San Francisco: The San Francisco General Hospital Foundation, 1999.

Blue, Rupert. "Fumigation of Vessels to Prevent the Spread of Plague." *Public Health Reports.* 28, no. 8 (1913): 346–47.

Book of Instruction for the Medical Inspection of Immigrants, Prepared by Direction of the Surgeon-General. Washington, DC: Government Printing Office, 1903.

Book of Instructions for the Medical Inspection of Aliens (rev. Jan. 18, 1910). Washington, DC: Government Printing Office, 1910.

Brechin, Gary. *Imperial San Francisco: Urban Power, Earthly Ruin.* Berkeley: University of California Press, 1999.

Bullough, William. *The Blind Boss & His City: Christopher Augustine Buckley and Nineteenth-Century San Francisco.* Berkeley: University of California Press, 1979.

Carrigan, Jo Ann. *The Saffron Scourge: A History of Yellow Fever in Louisiana, 1796–1905.* Lafayette: Center for Louisiana Studies, 1994.

Carter, Henry Rose. *Yellow Fever: An Epidemiological and Historical Study of Its Place of Origin.* Baltimore: Williams & Wilkins, 1931.

Chambers, J. S. *The Conquest of Cholera.* New York: Macmillan, 1938.

Chapin, Charles. "The Fetish of Disinfection." *Journal of the American Medical Association* 47, no. 8 (1906): 574–80.

Chapin, Charles. *The Sources and Modes of Infection,* 2nd ed. New York: John Wiley & Sons, 1916.

Chase, Marilyn. *The Barbary Plague: The Black Death in Victorian San Francisco.* New York: Random House, 2003.

Chase-Levenson, Alexander. "Early Nineteenth-Century Mediterranean Quarantine as a European System." In *Quarantine: Local and Global Histories,* edited by Alison Bashford. New York: Palgrave MacMillan, 2016, 43–44.

Clark, T., Passed Asst. Surg., and Passed Asst. Surg. J. W. Schereschewsky. *Trachoma: Its Character and Effects.* Washington, DC: Government Printing Office, 1907.

Cofer, Leland E. "A Word to Ship Captains about Quarantine: An Open Letter to Ship Captains." *Public Health Bulletin,* no. 55. Washington, DC: Government Printing Office, Jul. 1912.

Cofer, Leland E. "Maritime Quarantine." *Public Health Bulletin,* no. 34. Washington, DC: Government Printing Office, 1910: 1–64.

Coop, C. E., and H. M. Ginzburg. "The Revitalization of the Public Health Service Commissioned Corps." *Public Health Reports* 104, no. 2 (1989): 105–10.

Creel, R. H. "The Extension of Plague Infection of the Bubonic Type." *American Journal of Public Health* 6, no. 3 (1916): 191–221.

"Cyanogen Chloride Gas Mixture: Irritating Quality of New Fumigant Saves the Life of a Stowaway on Vessel Being Fumigated." *Public Health Reports* 39, no. 11 (1924): 529.

Davies, Andrea R. *Saving San Francisco: Relief and Recovery after the 1906 Disaster.* Philadelphia: Temple University Press, 2012.

Duffy, John, ed. *The Rudolph Matas History of Medicine in Louisiana.* Baton Rouge: Louisiana State University Press, 1915, vol 2.

Eager, J. M. *The Present Pandemic of Plague.* Washington, DC: Government Printing Office, 1908.

Eager, John Macauley. "The Early History of Quarantine: Origin of Sanitary Measures Directed Against Yellow Fever." *Yellow Fever Institute Bulletin* #12, Washington, DC: US Department of the Treasury, PHMHS, 1903.

Echenberg, Myron. *Plague Ports: The Global Urban Impact of Bubonic Plague, 1894–1901.* New York: New York University Press, 2007.

Editorial. "The Concealment of Plague Information." *Occidental Medical Times* 15, no. 6
     (1901): 215–18.

Editorial. *Occidental Medical Times* 14, no. 4 (1900): 121.

Editorial. *Pacific Medical and Surgical Journal* 25, no. 1 (1883): 381–82.

Editorial. *Pacific Medical and Surgical Journal* 31, no. 6 (1888): 347–49.

Editorial. *Pacific Medical and Surgical Journal* 31, no. 3 (1888): 155–59.

Editorial. *Pacific Medical and Surgical Journal* 31, no. 8 (1888): 474.

Editorial. *Science,* NS 13, no. 333 (1901): 761–65.

Editorial. *The Sanitarian* 13, 1884: 69.

Editorial. *The Sanitarian.* 9: 1881, 86–88.

Ellis, John H. *Yellow Fever and Public Health in the New South.* Lexington: University Press
     of Kentucky, 1992.

Fenner, Frank, Donald A. Henderson, Isao Arita, Zdenek Jezek, and Ivan D. Ladnyi.
     Smallpox and Its Eradication. Geneva: World Health Organization, 1988.

Findlay, G. M. "The First Recognized Epidemic of Yellow Fever." *Transactions of the Royal
     Society of Tropical Medicine* 35, no. 3 (1941): 143–54.

Flexner, Simon, F. G. Novy, and Lewellys F. Barker. *Report of the Commission Appointed
     by the Secretary of the Treasury for the Investigation of Plague in San Francisco.*
     Washington, DC: Government Printing Office, 1901.

Fradkin, Philip L. *The Great Earthquake and Firestorms of 1906: How San Francisco Nearly
     Destroyed Itself.* Berkeley: University of California Press, 2005.

Garrison, Fielding H. *An Introduction to the History of Medicine.* Philadelphia:
     W. B. Saunders, 1929.

Gates, Merrill E., ed. *Men of Mark in America.* Washington, DC: Men of Mark, 1906.

Gensini, Gian Franco, Yacoub, Magdi H., and Conti, Andrea A. "The Concept of
     Quarantine in History: From Plague to SARS." *Journal of Infection* 49, no. 4 (2004):
     257–61.

Gibbon, Henry. "The Variolous Epidemic in San Francisco in 1868." *Transactions of the
     American Medical Association* 20, 1869: 528–42.

Gold, Arthur. *The Divine Sarah: A Life of Sarah Bernhardt.* New York: Knopf, 1991.

Guerrant, Richard L., David H. Walker, and Peter F. Weller. *Tropical Infectious Disease:
     Principles, Pathogens, and Practice.* Philadelphia: Churchill Livingstone–Elsevier, 2006.

Hamilton, John B. "Quarantine Near New Orleans." *Weekly Abstract of Sanitary Reports* 3,
     no. 26((Jun). 29), 1888: 117–47.

Hamilton, John B. "Report on the Sanitation of Ships and Quarantine." *Annual Report of
     the Supervising Surgeon General of the United States Marine-Hospital Service, FY 1890.*
     Washington, DC: Government Printing Office, 85–95.

Harden, Victoria. *Inventing the NIH: Federal Biomedical Research Policy, 1887–1937.*
     Baltimore: Johns Hopkins University Press, 1986.

Harris, Henry. *California's Medical Story.* San Francisco: J W Stacey, 1932.

Harrison, Mark. *Contagion: How Commerce Has Spread Disease.* New Haven, CT: Yale
     University Press, 2012.

Hawgood, Barbara. "Waldemar Mordecai Haffkine, CIE (1860–1930): Prophylactic
     Vaccination against Cholera and Bubonic Plague in British India." *Journal of Medical
     Biography* 15, no. 1 (2007): 9–19.

Herrick, S.S. "Review of Smallpox in San Francisco from May 3, 1887 to March 21, 1888." *Pacific Medical Journal* 31, no. 4 (1888): 207–13.

Hirst, L. Fabian. *The Conquest of Plague: A Study of the Evolution of Epidemiology.* Oxford: Oxford University Press, 1953.

Holt, Joseph. "Address to the Louisiana State Board of Health." *New Orleans Medical and Surgical Journal* 11 (May 1884): 890–96.

Holt, Joseph. "The quarantine system of Louisiana–Methods of disinfection practiced." *Public Health Papers and Reports* 13, 1887: 161–87.

Holt, Joseph. *The New Quarantine System.* Reprinted in book form from *New Orleans Medical and Surgical Journal.* New Orleans, LA: New Orleans Medical Publishing Association, 1885.

Horlbeck, H. B. "Maritime Sanitation at Ports of Arrival." *Public Health Papers and Reports* 16, 1890: 110–25.

Howard, John. *An Account of the Principle Lazzarettos in Europe; with Various Papers Relative to the Plague; Together with Further Observations on Some Foreign Prisons and Hospitals; and Additional Remarks on the Present State of Those in Great Britain and Ireland.* London: William Eyres, 1789.

Howard-Jones, Norman. *The Scientific Background of the International Sanitary Conferences, 1851–1938.* Geneva: World Health Organization, 1975.

Humphreys, Margaret. *Yellow Fever and the South.* Baltimore: Johns Hopkins University Press, 1992.

Ileto, Reynaldo C. "Cholera and the Origins of the American Sanitary Order in the Philippines," in *Imperial Medicine and Indigenous Societies,* edited by David Arnold, 125–48. New York: Manchester University Press, 1988.

Ireland, M. W., and F. W. Weed, in *The Medical Department of the United States Army in the World War, vol. 5: Military Hospitals in the United States.* Washington, DC: Government Printing Office, 1923.

Issel, William, and Robert W. Cherney. *San Francisco, 1865–1932: Politics, Power, and Urban Development.* Berkeley: University of California Press, 1986.

Ji-Hye. "The 'Oriental' Problem: Trachoma and Asian Immigrants in the United States, 1897–1910." *Korean Journal of Medical History* 23, no. 3 (2014): 573–603.

Jones, Guy P. "Thomas Logan, MD, Organizer of California State Board of Health and a Co-founder of the California Medical Association." *California and Western Medicine* 63, no. 1 (1945): 6–10.

Kalisch, Philip. "The Black Death in Chinatown: Plague and Politics in San Francisco 1900–1904." *Arizona and the West* 14, no. 2 (1972): 113–36.

Kazanjian, Powel. "Frederick Novy and the 1901 San Francisco Plague Commission Investigation." *Clinical Infectious Diseases* 55, no. 10 (2012): 1373–78.

Koch, Robert. "Die Aetiologie der Milzbrand-Krankheit, Begründet auf die Entwicklungsgeschichte des Bacillus Anthracis." *Beiträge zur Biologie der Pflanzen* 2, 1876: 277–310.

Kraut, Alan M. *Silent Travelers: Germs, Genes, and the "Immigration Menace."* Baltimore: Johns Hopkins University Press, 1994.

Lai, H. M. "Island of Immortals: Chinese Immigrants and the Angel Island Immigration Station." *California History* 57, no. 1 (1978): 88–103.

Lee, Erika, and Judy Yung. *Angel Island: Immigrant Gateway to America.* New York: Oxford University Press, 2010.

Lee, Erika. *At America's Gates: Chinese Immigration During the Exclusion Era, 1882–1943.* Chapel Hill: University of North Carolina Press, 2005.

Lewis, Oscar. *San Francisco: Mission to Metropolis.* Berkeley: Howell-North Books, 1966.

Link, Vernon B. "The New Orleans Epidemics." *A History of Plague in the United States of America, chap. 5.* Public Health Monograph #26. Washington, DC: Government Printing Office, 1955.

Lipson, L. G. "Plague in San Francisco: The United States Marine Hospital Service Commission to Study the Existence of Plague in San Francisco." *Annals of Internal Medicine* 77, no. 2 (1972): 303–110.

Lister, Joseph. "Illustrations of the Antiseptic System of Treatment in Surgery." *The Lancet* Nov. 30, 1867: 668–69.

Lucaccini, L. F. "The Public Health Service on Angel Island." *Public health Reports* 111, no. 1 (1996): 92–94.

Lyman, George D. "The Beginnings of California's Medical History." *California and Western Medicine* 23, no. 5 (1925): 561–76.

MacGillivray, Don. *Captain Alex MacLean: Jack London's Sea Wolf.* Vancouver, BC: University of British Columbia Press, 2008.

Mandell, Gerald L., John E. Bennett, and Raphael Dolin. *Principles and Practice of Infectious Diseases,* 5th ed. Philadelphia: Churchill Livingstone, 2000.

Markel, Howard. "The Eyes Have it: Trachoma, the Perception of Disease, the United States Public Health Service, and the American Jewish Immigration Experience." *Bulletin of the History of Medicine* 74, no. 3 (2000): 525–60.

Matovinovic, Josip. "A Short History of Quarantine." *University of Michigan Medical Center Journal* 35, no. 4 (1969): 224–28.

McGloin, John B. *San Francisco: The Story of a City.* San Rafael, CA: Presidio Press, 1978.

Meyer, K. F. "The Ecology of Psittacosis and Ornithosis." *Medicine* 21, no. 2 (1942): 175–206.

Meyer, K. F., Dan C. Cavanaugh, Peter J. Bartelloni, and John D. Marshall, Jr. "Plague Immunization. I. Past and Present Trends." *Journal of Infectious Diseases* 129, suppl (1974): S13–S18.

Michael, J. M. "The National Board of Health." *Public Health Reports* 126, no. 1 (2011): 123–29.

Miller, Stuart Creighton. *The Unwelcome Immigrant: The American Image of the Chinese, 1785–1882.* Berkeley: University of California Press, 1969.

"Milton Joseph Rosenau." *American Journal of Public Health* 36, no. 5 (1936): 530–31.

Mohr, James C. *Plague and Fire: Battling Black Death and the 1900 Burning of Honolulu's Chinatown.* New York: Oxford University Press, 2005.

Moore, Sarah J. *Empire on Display: San Francisco's Panama-Pacific International Exposition of 1915.* Norman: University of Oklahoma Press, 2013.

Morens, David M., and Anthony S. Fauci. "The Forgotten Forefather: Joseph James Kinyoun and the Founding of the National Institutes of Health." mBio 3, no. 4 (2012): 139–12.

Mullan, Fitzhugh. *Plagues and Politics: The Story of the United States Public Health Service.* New York: Basic Books, Inc, 1989.

Muscatin, Doris. *Old San Francisco: The Biography of a City from Early Days to the Earthquake.* New York: G.P. Putnam's Sons, 1975.

Neu, Charles E. *An Unusual Friendship: Theodore Roosevelt and Japan, 1906–1909.* Cambridge: Harvard University Press, 1967.

New York Academy of Medicine, Public Health, Hospital, and Budget Committee. "Quarantine in the Maritime Cities of the United States." *Journal of the American Medical Association* 60, no. 4 (1913): 194–200.

Perry, Alfred. "Effectual External Sanitary Regulations Without Delay to Commerce." *Public Health Reports and Papers.* New York: Hurd and Houghton, 1873, 437–40.

Perry, Alfred. "Quarantine Without Obstruction to Commerce." *New Orleans Medical and Surgical Journal,* N. S. 1, no. 1 (1874): 567–72.

Perry, Alfred. "Report of Sanitary Inspector, Fourth District." *Annual Report of the Board of Health to the General Assembly of Louisiana,* December 31st, 1872. New Orleans: Board of Health, 1873: 92–99.

Perry, Alfred. "Report of Sanitary Inspector, Fourth District." *Annual Report of the Board of Health to the General Assembly of Louisiana,* December 31st, 1873. New Orleans: Board of Health, 1874, 188–93.

Phelps, Alonzo. *Contemporary Biography of California's Representative Men.* San Francisco: A L Bancroft, 1881.

Platzer, Richard F. "Evaluation of Therapeutic agents in Plague." *U. S. Naval Medical Bulletin* 46, no. 11 (1946): 1674–89.

Pollitzer, R. *Cholera.* Geneva: World Health Organization, 1959.

Public Health and Marine Hospital Service (PHMHS). Book of Instructions for the Medical Inspection of Aliens (rev. Jan. 18, 1910). Washington, DC: US Government Printing Office, 1910.

Public Health, Hospital, and Budget Committee of the New York Academy of Medicine. "Quarantine in the Maritime Cities of the United States." *Journal of the American Medical Association* 60, no. 3 (1913):194–200.

Ralston, John C. *This Date in San Francisco: 366 Days in the History of Our Beloved Fascinating City.* Mountain View, CA: RIW Publishing, 2001.

Rauch, John H. *Report of an inspection of the Atlantic and Gulf Quarantines between the St. Lawrence and Rio Grande.* Springfield: Illinois State Board of Health, 1886.

Reuther, Walter, E. Clair Calavan, and Glenn E. Carman, eds. *The Citrus Industry,* 5, Oakland: Division of Agriculture and Natural Resources, University of California, 1989.

Ridlon, J. R. "Some Aspects of Ship Fumigation." *Public Health Reports* 46, no. 27 (1931): 1572–78.

Risse, Guenther B. *Plague, Fear, and Politics in San Francisco's Chinatown.* Baltimore: Johns Hopkins University Press, 2012.

Roberts, N. "Fumigation of the USS *Tennessee* by the Cyanide Method." *United States Naval Medical Bulletin* 10, no. 2 (1916): 296–300.

Rosen, George. *A History of Public Health, expanded edition.* Baltimore: Johns Hopkins University Press, 1993.

Rosenberg, Charles E. *The Cholera Years*. Chicago: University of Chicago Press,1962.

Salomon, Lucien F. "The Louisiana Quarantine System and its Contemplated Improvement." *Public Health Papers and Reports* 14, 1888: 110–15.

Salyer, Lucy E. *Laws Harsh as Tigers*. Chapel Hill: University of North Carolina Press, 1995.

Sehdev, Paul S. "The Origin of Quarantine." *Clinical Infectious Diseases* 35, no. 9 (2002): 1071–72.

"Ship Fumigation: Preliminary Report of the Board Appointed by the Surgeon General to Investigate the Subject of Fumigation of Ships." *Public Health Reports* 37, no. 44 (1922): 2744–48.

Soennichsen, John. *Miwoks to Missiles: A History of Angel Island*. Tiburon, CA: Angel Island Association, 2005.

Spence, Jonathan. *The Search for Modern China*. New York: W.W. Norton, 1990.

Starr, Kevin. *Golden Gate: The Life and Times of America's Greatest Bridge*. New York: Bloomsbury Press, 2010.

Sternberg, George M. *Report on the Etiology and Prevention of Yellow Fever*. Washington, DC: Government Printing Office, 1890.

Stiles, Charles Wardell. "A Brief Review of Certain Phases of Hookworm Disease." In *Transactions of the Seventh Annual Conference of State and Territorial Health Officers with the United States Public Health and Marine-Hospital Service June 2, 1909*, 59–62. Washington, DC: Government Printing Office, 1910.

Stuard, Susan Mosher. *A State of Deference: Ragusa/Dubrovnik in the Medieval Centuries*. Philadelphia: Univ. of Pennsylvania Press, 1992.

Summers, William. *The Great Manchurian Plague of 1910–1911: The Geopolitics of an Epidemic Disease*. New Haven, CT: Yale University Press, 2012.

Swartz, Morton N. "Bacterial Meningitis–A View of the Past 90 Years." *New England Journal of Medicine* 351, no. 18 (2004): 1826–28.

"The New Orleans Epidemics." In *USPHS Public Health Monograph* #26, chap. 6. Washington, DC: Government Printing Office, 1955, 44.

Todd, Frank. M., ed. *Eradicating Plague from San Francisco: Report of the Citizen's Health Committee and an Account of its Work*. San Francisco: C. A. Murdock, 1909.

Toogood, Anna Coxe. *A Civil History of Golden Gate National Recreation Area and Point Reyes National Seashore*. Washington, DC: Historic Preservation Branch, National Park Service, US Department of the Interior, 1980.

Tower, Paul. "The History of Trachoma: Its Military and Sociological Implications." *Archives of Ophthalmology* 69, no. 1 (1963): 123–30.

"Trachoma among Immigrants." *New York Medical Journal* 93, no. 17 (1911): 835.

Trauner, Joan B. "The Chinese as Medical Scapegoats in San Francisco, 1870–1905." *California History* 57, no. 1 (1978): 70–87.

Waksman, Selman A. *The Brilliant and Tragic Life of W. M. W. Haffkine, Bacteriologist*. New Brunswick, NJ: Rutgers University Press, 1964.

Wayson, N. E. "Clonorchis Investigations: A Summary of Surveys and Experiments to Determine Whether Clonorchiasis May be Disseminated in the Pacific Slope of the United States." *Public Health Reports* 42, no. 51 (1927): 3129–35.

Wendt, Edmund Charles, ed. *A Treatise on Asiatic Cholera*. New York: William Wood, 1885.

Williams, Ralph C. *The United States Public Health Service*. Washington, DC:
Commissioned Officers Association of the United States Public Health Service, 1951.

Winchester, Simon. *A Crack in the Edge of the World: America and the Great California
Earthquake of 1906*. New York: Harper Collins, 2005.

Winslow, Charles-Edward Amory. *The Conquest of Epidemic Disease: A Chapter in the
History of Ideas*. Princeton, NJ: Princeton University Press, 1943.

Wong, Yu Fong. *Historical Review of Clonorchiasis*. San Francisco: Chinese Six Companies,
1927.

Woodworth, John M. "The General Subject of Quarantine with Special Reference to
Cholera and Yellow Fever," in *Transactions of the International Medical Congress of
Philadelphia of 1876*, edited by John Ashhurst. Philadelphia: International Medical
Congress, 1877: 1059.

Wu, Lien-the. *Plague Fighter: The Autobiography of a Modern Chinese Physician*. Cambridge:
W. Heffer & Sons, 1959.

Ziegler, Philip. *The Black Death*. New York: John Day Co, 1969.

INTERNET SOURCES

"An Act to Prohibit the Coming of Chinese Laborers to the United States." 1888. 50th
Congress, Session I, Chap. 1015, p 476. https://college.cengage.com/history/ayers
_primary_sources/prohibitcoming_chinese_laborers.htm

"An Act to Prevent the Introduction of Contagious Diseases from one State to Another."
Mar. 27, 1890. at:https://tile.loc.gov/storage-services/service/ll/llsl//llsl-c51/llsl-c51.pdf,
31-32.

"An Act to Regulate the Immigration of Aliens into the United States," Mar. 3, 1903.
Statutes at Large of the United States of America from November 1902 to March 1905,
chap. 1012, 1213–22. https://tile.loc.gov/storage-services/service/ll/llsl//llsl-c57/llsl-c57
.pdf; quotes on 1214.

"An Act to regulate the immigration of aliens to, and the residence of aliens in, the
United States." Record of 64th Congress, Session II, Chap 29, February 5th, 1917.
Section 16. https://curiosity.lib.harvard.edu/immigration-to-the-united-states-1789
–1930/catalog/39–990100032410203941

Centers for Disease Control and Prevention article. https://www.cdc.gov/tuskegee
/timeline.htm

Chinese Exclusion Act of 1882. https://www.ourdocuments.gov/doc.php?doc=47

"A History of UCSF: R. Beverly Cole." University of California San Francisco website.
http://history.library.ucsf.edu/cole.html

Influenza epidemic: an excellent account of the epidemic, prepared by the University
of Michigan Center for the History of Medicine. http://www.influenzaarchive.org
/cities/city-sanfrancisco.html#

Long, Esmond R. Frederick George Novy, 1864–1957: A Biographical Memoir,
Washington DC.: National Academy of Sciences, 1959. http://www.nasonline.org
/publications/biographical-memoirs/memoir-pdfs/novy-frederick.pdf

Morens, David M. and Anthony S. Fauci. "The Forgotten Forefather: Joseph James Kinyoun and the Founding of the National Institutes of Health." mBio 3, no. 4 (2012): e00139–12. Published online 2012 Jun 26. DOI: 10.1128/mBio.00139–12, https://journals.asm.org/doi/10.1128/mBio.00139–12

Plague in Venice: National Geographic News, Aug. 29, 2007. http://news.national geographic.com/news/2007/08/070829-venice-plague.html

Risse, Guenter B. "Science Contested: Bacteriologists and Bubonic Plague in San Francisco." Unpublished lecture, Conference on the Laboratory in 20th Century Medicine: Historical Perspectives, University of California, San Francisco, Jan. 22, 1998. at https://www.researchgate.net/publication/301765393_Science_Contested _Bacteriologists_and_Bubonic_Plague_in_San_Francisco

Surgeon General Website (Wyman). http://wayback.archive-it.org/3929/20171201191736 /https://www.surgeongeneral.gov/about/previous/biowyman.html

Surgeon General Website (Cumming). http://wayback.archive-it.org/3929/20171201191738 /https://www.surgeongeneral.gov/about/previous/biocumming.html

Surgeon General, Office of, US Department of Health and Human Services (Rupert Blue). https://web.archive.org/web/20080916014409/http://surgeongeneral.gov/about /previous/bioblue.htm

"U.S. Public Health Service Commissioned Corps: History." https://web.archive.org/web /20121020040704/http://www.usphs.gov/aboutus/history.aspx

Woods, Arnold. "Spanish Flu in SF: A Closer Look." Open SF History, March, 2020. https://opensfhistory.org/news/2020/03/14/spanish-flu-in-sf-a-closer-look/

Index

Act to Regulate the Immigration of Aliens into the United States of 1903, 79

adrenalin, 82

Aedes mosquito, 14–15, 74–75

Alcatraz Island, x, 3, 29

American Cyanamid Company, 113

American Expeditionary Force, 126. *See also* US Army

American Medical Association, 26, 30

American Public Health Association, 18, 22–23, 135

amoebas, 106

anarchists, 79

Angel Island, ix, x, 11; as California State Park and, 132; fires and, 41, 51, 129, 137; history of, 28–29; landscape and, xi, 3, 28, 33; lighthouse and, 131; museum and, 132, 137; proposed as quarantine site and, x, 28, 30, 33; quarry and, 29; rats and, 101–2; US Army and, 29, 76, 86, 101, 129, 131. *See also* US Immigration Service Station

Angel Island Quarantine Station, ix–x, 11, 99; closing and, 131–32, 133, 136; coming to the end of its use and, 109–10, 123, 124, 127–28, 129, 130, 131–32; conditions and, xi, 34, 39, 41, 43, 44, 45–46, 47, 48–50, 83–87, 100–104, 127, 137; flu epidemic and, 109; MHS establishment of and, x, 23, 24, 30, 33, 39; opening and, ix, x, xii, 13, 14–15, 16, 17, 33–34, 41, 133; San Francisco earthquake and, 88–89, 157n2; US Army and, 40, 41, 43, 44, 46, 49, 84, 86, 101, 127, 131; US Immigration Service Station and, xi, 102, 105–7, 129,

130; weather and, 43, 44, 45, 84–85, 89, 96–97, 101; World War I and, 108. *See also* Marine Hospital Service (MHS); Public Health and Marine Hospital Service (PHMHS); Public Health Service

Angel Island Quarantine Station medical officers, 51, 53–54, 90; administration and, 41, 44, 45–46, 83, 86–87, 103; first serving and, xii, 33, 35, 36, 39, 40; later work and, 134–35; living conditions and, 84, 130, 133; medical examinations and, 50–51; medical examinations for US Immigration Service and, xi, 77–78, 79–82, 94, 99, 105–7, 127, 130; as quarantine officer and, 58, 59–62, 68–69, 71–72, 73, 77–78, 87, 133, 151–52n2; ship inspections and, 55, 56–57, 58–60, 71; Spanish-American War and, 73, 74

Angel Island Quarantine Station operations, 12, 17, 136; contagious disease vigilance and, 51, 73, 74, 76–77, 78, 87, 90, 111, 123, 132, 133; disinfecting and, 33, 34, 39, 43, 44, 47, 49–50, 52, 57, 58, 59, 60, 77, 83, 100, 108, 124, 132; electricity and, 41, 49, 85, 101; fees and, 39, 43, 46, 47, 52–53, 77; fumigation of buildings and, 43, 44, 84; funding and, 32, 34, 36, 40, 41, 46, 49, 86, 133; laboratory and, 54, 57, 91, 100, 104, 106; lacking supplies and, 34, 35, 39–40, 46, 95; local vs. federal operation and, 41–42, 46, 52–53, 54–58; MHS running of and, 41–42, 48, 52; overseas bills of health and, 51, 56, 77, 78, 104, 124; pharmacy and, 103; sewage disposal and, 34, 39,

About the Author

John Gordon Frierson was engaged in the practice of internal medicine and infectious diseases in Oakland, California, for many years. He is Emeritus Clinical Professor in the Department of Medicine at the University of California San Francisco. Now retired, he devotes time to his longstanding interest in the history of medicine and publishes a blog on the subject. He currently lives in Palo Alto, California.